"Excellent . . . Gogs Gagnon provides very keen observations throughout, from the early stages to treatment and recovery. It's clear he has done a lot of research on the topic."

— Ted Butterfield, past Chair
Prostate Cancer Foundation BC
a long-term 'living with prostate cancer patient'

"As a medical practitioner that treats prostate cancer, it was invaluable to read a patient's journey from diagnosis to treatment and beyond — an excellent read for anyone impacted by this disease."

— Dr. Aaron Clark, MD, FRCSC
Urologist
North Island Urology, Courtenay, BC

"Gagnon's musings are enhanced with his situational humor, balancing the seriousness of his diagnosis. Others going through these stages will be comforted."

— Dr. Michael A. Geffin, MD
Chief Medical Officer, Director, Advanced Prostate Cancer Care
Greater Boston Urology, Dedham, Massachusetts

"This is such an insightful and educational story. Any man who has been diagnosed with prostate cancer should read this book early in his journey."

— Connie Degenstein, BScN, RN
Resource Nurse
Island Prostate Centre, Victoria, BC

"I found myself crying, laughing and cheering . . . I wish this book had been available when my husband and I first received the frightening news he had prostate cancer."

— Glenda Standeven, inspirational speaker and bone cancer survivor
Author of *What Men Won't Talk About . . . And Women need to Know:
A Woman's Perspective on Prostate Cancer*

"Insightful, sensitive and helpful . . . The subject of cancer is complex, but this book manages to present sufficient detail for readers to come away more knowledgeable."

— Dr. Daniela Chifor, MD, CCFP
Family Physician, Clinical Instructor
University of British Columbia

"Gogs Gagnon's honesty and humility offers all men diagnosed with prostate cancer the grounding and confidence they will need to seek out the doctors and treatments that are best for them and to take control of their prostate cancer journey."

— Brian Lynch, CEO
Nuada Medical Prostate Experts
Abingdon, Oxfordshire, UK

"I truly believe that Gogs Gagnon's research and personal understanding of the disease will help others, whether they are facing prostate cancer themselves, or are simply curious about it."

— Arden Bagni
Daughter of a prostate cancer survivor

"This book gives much-needed insight from a patient's aspect, and Gogs' description of his experience is a wonderful read."

— Linda Hoetger, Social Media Ambassador
ZERO — The End of Prostate Cancer
Canal Winchester, Ohio

"An informative account of a journey that too many of us make."

— Joe Dahoy
Chair, Prostate Cancer Support Group, Campbell River, Canada
Executive Member, Prostate Cancer Foundation BC

"A must read for anyone (and their families) who is given the diagnosis of cancer."

— Zosia Ettenberg, CEO
Langley Pos-Abilities Society, BC
Breast cancer survivor and author of *Cancer — I Won!*

"Inspirational . . . Gagnon addresses every question you could imagine, including all the questions that you may even be afraid to speak to your doctor about."

— Michael Aikins, Chief Administrative Officer
The Views at St. Joseph's, Comox, BC

"*Prostate Cancer Strikes* is informative, candid and told with wisdom and true emotion."

— Amanda Walz
Daughter of a breast cancer survivor

Prostate Cancer Strikes

Prostate Cancer Strikes
Navigating The Storm

Gogs Gagnon

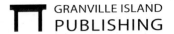

GRANVILLE ISLAND
PUBLISHING

Publisher's Cataloging-in-Publication Data

Names: Gagnon, Gogs, author.
Title: Prostate cancer strikes : navigating the storm / Gogs Gagnon.
Description: Vancouver, BC: Granville Island Publishing Ltd., 2019.
Identifiers: ISBN 978-1-926991-94-8 (pbk.) | 978-1-926991-97-9 (e-book)
Subjects: LCSH Gagnon, Gogs — Health. | Prostate — Cancer — Patients — Canada — Biography. | Prostate — Cancer — Popular works. | Men — Health and hygiene. |
BISAC HEALTH & FITNESS / Diseases / Cancer
HEALTH & FITNESS / Men's Health
Classification: LCC RC280.P7 .G34 2019 | DDC 616.99/463 — dc23

Book editor: Jen Groundwater
Book designer: Omar Gallegos
Proofreader: Rebecca Coates
Cover image: Courtesy of Pixabay.com
Author photo: Sharon Snider

Granville Island Publishing Ltd.
212 – 1656 Duranleau St.
Vancouver, BC, Canada V6H 3S4

604-688-0320 / 1-877-688-0320
info@granvilleislandpublishing.com
www.granvilleislandpublishing.com

Printed in Canada on recycled paper

This book is dedicated to all who have lived and are living with prostate cancer, their families and loved ones, and the medical professionals involved. My thoughts are with you.

CONTENTS

Acknowledgements

First and foremost, I thank my wife, Mary, for her love and support. She stood by my side throughout diagnosis, surgery and recovery, and demonstrated the utmost patience even while I spent many long hours writing this memoir and leaving her in isolation. I'm extremely fortunate to have her in my life, and I love her with all my heart and soul.

With much affection and love, I'm indebted to my children, Stacey, Alex and Jenn, who helped me tremendously with daily tasks during recovery. They sprang into action when I needed them most, and I'm proud to be their dad.

I'm eternally grateful and give thanks to my relatives, friends and neighbours who provided a great deal of comfort and strength through conversation and humour. They helped distract my mind from worry.

With immense respect and admiration, my wife and I express our most sincere thanks to the urologist/ surgeon and the surgical team at St. Joseph's General

Hospital. Their knowledge, patience and calm nature in the face of our endless barrage of questions put us at ease. We shall be forever grateful for their help and support.

With much appreciation, I would like to recognize the nurses who cared for me, including the student nurses and their instructor from North Island College. They were very caring, warm, professional and exceptional people who went the extra mile to provide excellent care and support during my stay in the hospital.

With tremendous gratitude and a warm heart, I give thanks to my cousin, mentors and friends who gave their time to provide valuable feedback and encouraged me to keep on writing.

A very special thank you to Granville Island Publishing and their phenomenal team who helped me tremendously. I want to acknowledge the following people; Jo Blackmore, who encouraged me from the beginning and always challenged me to do better by asking tough questions to ensure I worked hard to provide my best. Daniel Colmont, who consistently provided outstanding support and assistance. Jen Groundwater, a professional editor who was an absolute pleasure to work with and added significant value. Omar Gallegos, an expert book designer with an eye for perfection. David Litvak, a publicist who generated press coverage and helped prepare me for interviews. Rebecca Coates, a proofreader with excellent focus and attention to detail who polished and made the final product shine. Sam Margolis, who designed and developed a website that makes me proud. And finally, Conni Vogelfänger, an international marketer who helped raise global awareness. Writing this memoir was a surreal process, and required a lot more time and energy than I ever imagined. Because of the efforts, support and encouragement of Granville Island Publishing and their team, I found the whole experience enriching, and rewarding. I now have a legacy that I'm incredibly proud to pass on to help others impacted by this devastating disease.

A special shout-out to David Conn, who encouraged me to broaden the original manuscript to reach and inform more readers.

A heartfelt thank you to Michelle, a personal trainer who was instrumental in helping me get back into the gym with confidence. She has revived the spirit of my youth and instilled me with determination to continue on the road to achieving my fitness and nutrition goals.

I want to thank *everyone* who had ever said a kind word to me. Know that you have been a positive influence in my life.

Last but not least, I'm thankful for my two dogs, Maya and Nelly, for their unconditional love. They've taught me to slow down and enjoy the simple things in life, such as walking, playing, eating, sleeping and most importantly, connecting with people.

FOREWORD

IN 2017, Comox Valley software programmer Gogs Gagnon was diagnosed with prostate cancer. He was one of 21,300 Canadian men to get that jarring news. To him, in seemingly healthy middle age, it was a life-changing bolt from the blue.

Most men who are diagnosed deal with it as best they can. They inform their families and rapidly learn about the disease. They take stock and do a bit of soul-searching. They consult doctors and choose a medical treatment, or surveillance of the cancer. Most diagnosed men do receive treatment, and then try to get on with their lives.

Gogs did all that and more. He wrote this account of his own bout with prostate cancer in British Columbia. It's a record of his experiences and reactions as a man, husband, father and patient. While the content is often serious, he slips in quite a bit of humour — such as imagined discussions among his organs. Pop culture quotes offer a philosophical counterpoint. He comes across as a smart, social guy people would like to know.

While describing his diagnosis, treatment and recovery in detail, Gogs includes information for readers having their own prostate cancer experiences. There's a bibliography of websites and other informative books to aid further research.

As a veteran writer and a prostate cancer survivor, I got involved when the publisher asked me to look over Gogs' initial manuscript. I had reviewed many recent prostate cancer books written for the public, and was leery of personal testimonies by patients. However, I found Gogs' narrative compelling. He kept the story clear, learned as he went, and laid out his thoughts and feelings at each stage. To reach and inform more readers, I suggested broadening the scope of the book beyond detailing his process. He took up that suggestion and fulfilled it completely, also adding some advice for others from his voyage "navigating the storm."

So here, newly diagnosed patients and their families, anxious for some authentic yet reader-friendly information, can get a sense of what they may be dealing with. Gogs is a fine guide.

David R. Conn
Freelance researcher, writer, editor,
and prostate cancer survivor

CHAPTER ONE

IN THE BEGINNING

If a man dwells on the past, then he robs the present. But if a man ignores the past, he may rob the future. The seeds of our destiny are nurtured by the roots of our past.

— Master Po, speaking to Caine
    Dialogue from the TV series *Kung Fu*, "The Tide" episode, 1973

INTRODUCTION

MY NAME IS GOGS GAGNON, and on March 6, 2017, I was diagnosed with prostate cancer at the age of 57. Less than two months later, on May 1, I was on the table for three hours, undergoing radical prostatectomy surgery. The surgeons removed my entire prostate, seminal vesicles, some nearby lymph nodes, some surrounding tissue and part of my urethra.

After some serious thought, I have decided to share my prostate cancer story on a personal level. In these pages, I share intimate details of my diagnosis, surgery and recovery. It is my intent to capture what it was like and how it felt every step of the way, including what I should have done differently, as seen in hindsight through the lens of my newfound knowledge and experience.

I sincerely hope my story provides value to you and your loved ones and empowers you to become your own health advocate. May it inspire you to stay positive and research your options, and encourage you to speak with multiple medical professionals regarding your specific case. Beware: some parts contain mature content that won't be suitable for all audiences.

Background

The year was 2012, and I considered myself in good health and excellent physical condition. After all, I had ridden my bike to and from work for the past 25 years, trained in martial arts four to five days a week and hit the gym three to four times a week. I wasn't on any prescription medication and had no medical issues. I've never smoked or used street drugs and have only the odd drink on special occasions. Overall, I was in the best shape of my life.

I attribute this to the early days of my childhood. I have extremely fond memories of growing up near the town of Maillardville, a French community on the south slope of Coquitlam, BC. It was the largest francophone centre west of Manitoba and had a population of about 55,000 people between the years 1959 and the mid-1970s — a time long before the internet, cell phones and personal computers.

Everybody knew each other on our street, and it was not uncommon to go inside a neighbour's house to use the washroom or to find something to eat. I lived next door to my relatives, the McRobb family, and spent most of the time with my cousin Bruce. In summer, we'd spend most days outside with the neighbourhood kids, morning to night, playing games such as street hockey, baseball and marbles, riding our bikes and building tree forts. In winter, we'd spend the day sledding, building snow forts and having snowball fights. On rainy days, we'd play board games or read *Popular Mechanics*, *Popular Science* and comic books. Basically, no matter the weather, there was always something to do. My core values and beliefs are heavily influenced by this time period.

My father[1] was a self-taught tradesman who often worked multiple jobs to support the family. He specialized in cement and plaster and had a passion for his craft. He often provided extremely creative solutions to problems others told him could not be solved — he would always find a way. Once, he was told he couldn't attach bricks to a concrete retaining wall. After some thought, he applied a special coating of cement and,

---

1   Henry "Allan" Gagnon, born in Bonnyville, Alberta in 1933. His mother, Lena Rose Gagnon (née Marcoux), was also from Bonnyville and his father, Ernest Gagnon, was from Québec City, Québec.

using string and a level, he etched vertical and horizontal lines to make the surface look like bricks. Once dried and painted red with a roller, it looked exactly like a brick wall. It's still standing to this day.

In his youth, my father was a boxer and a hockey player who wore his hair in a ducktail and enjoyed street racing. His philosophy was simple: work hard, play hard, don't let anyone tell you what you can't do, stand on your own two feet and don't let people push you around. Overall, my father was a straight shooter, full of confidence, with a never-give-up attitude.

When I was 12 years old, my father taught me how to mix cement and plaster and put me to work. We didn't have a cement mixer at the time and mixed everything by hand. I remember the hard work of mixing, pushing heavy wheelbarrows on narrow planks, carrying countless buckets of plaster up ladders and across scaffoldings, and keeping the work area and tools spotlessly clean.

He taught me to realize you had done a great job when there was no evidence any work had been done. This meant that in addition to cleaning up the work area and putting away the tools, the renovation was so seamless that only you knew where the work had been done. Although it was hard work and long hours, there was no better reward and feeling than to sit back and admire the end results.

In addition to learning the valuable lesson that hard work is its own reward, my father taught me his boxing skills so I could defend myself. Not only had he fought in the ring in his youth, he had also fought in the streets. Knowing that my father had such skills piqued my interest, as there was always a fight after school in the parking lot or behind the church. I remember having to run home at the end of class to avoid getting a beating. After a few lessons, my self-esteem and confidence improved to a point where I learned how to avoid the fights and no longer had to run away. The extra confidence alone was enough for the bullies at school to leave me alone.

A short time later, my interest in boxing gave way to a fascination with other martial arts after the movie *Enter the Dragon* with Bruce Lee hit the big screen in 1973. My younger brother, David, and I must have watched the movie dozens of times. We knew every scene, every move and all of the dialogue. Together, we'd rehearse the fight scenes and imitate the voices of all the actors. Our father recognized our enthusiasm and made us every weapon in the movie.

Over the years, David trained in many different martial-arts styles — later in life, he lived in Japan for ten years to study ninjutsu. I pursued martial arts part-time and continued to work with my father, mixing cement and plaster for many years, until our parents split up for a short time in the early part of 1977.

Our mother moved us to Edmonton, Alberta, into a townhouse complex that was close to our sister Joanne and her husband, and within one week she found a job as a cleaner at a local hospital. To keep up our education, she enrolled us in nearby schools. For me, it was bad timing, as it was just a few months before Grade 12 graduation. I didn't know anybody and had little interest in going. Needless to say, I didn't learn much and graduated at the bottom of the class. I told myself that I was never going to school again.

Then something unexpected happened. Our father came to visit later that same year and said he had gotten a job in Victoria, BC (Vancouver Island) working as a tradesmen supervisor for the BC government. After a lengthy talk, our parents decided to get back together, and we all moved to Victoria. The best part came when, a short time later, Joanne and her husband also moved to Victoria. Joanne and I shared a special bond and were extremely close, and I was over the moon to know we would once again live in the same city.

After the move, I found work at McDonald's for a short period and then as a janitor at a local hospital, and was very content and happy, with no plans or desire to leave. That is, until I purchased a TI-59 programmable calculator with a magnetic card reader in 1979. Little did I know at the time that this calculator was about to change my life. That was the beginning of my interest in technology, which, after I coded my first program, turned into an obsession.

In 1980, I purchased an Apple IIe computer, quit my job, enrolled at Camosun College and took every computer course available. Computers fascinated me, and I spent every waking hour reading and learning how to develop code. Recognizing the need for another computer, my father bought me a Kaypro II and encouraged me to continue my studies. My obsession soon turned to passion, and I found myself in the computer lab programming away on New Year's

Eve. I didn't notice when the clock struck midnight. For me, it was just another day to write code.

For someone who'd declared that they were never going to school again, I was doing incredibly well, with a thirst for more knowledge, achieving straight A's. That was, until I met my future wife, Mary, in 1982. We instantly fell in love and were married four months later. Even though my grades slid a bit due to my new love interest, I still managed to graduate at the top of my class in 1983 with a diploma of technology in computer science and technical applications.

For the first few years, I developed games for Apple Computer and utility software for IBM and independently developed and marketed one of the first BC income tax programs approved by Revenue Canada that didn't require the use of pre-printed forms. In 1985, I took a job as a computer programmer for the BC government. Thirty years later, I retired to work as a part-time contractor.

Even after all these years as a computer programmer, I still especially enjoy complex programming issues that require extremely creative solutions to solve.

I live for these issues, which remind me of my father and his determination always to find a way and to never give up. Solving such complex matters provides me with a natural high, both at the time and when I recall the situation years later. Again, it's admiring the results of your work that gives the highest reward.

Although I didn't follow in the footsteps of my father as a tradesman, I've adopted his philosophies in life, his passion for work and the same can-do and never-give-up attitude. Today, my eighty-four-year old father is a professional ballroom dancer and is in good health.[2]

When it comes to eating, I haven't scored as well and continue to struggle to eat healthily. During my youth, I ate tons of sweets, including buckets of pudding, bowls of raw cookie dough, cake batter, icing, tons of chocolate and my all-time favourite: a whole bag of candy bought at the corner store for just 25 cents. To buy another bag of candy, all I needed to do was collect enough pop bottles from around the neighbourhood. Such overindulgences continued into my adult life.

All this talk of eating sweets fondly reminds me of my mother.[3] In my youth, there was always something to eat at our house. She had a passion for baking, reading and entertaining many friends and family throughout the year. She was also known for her quick wit and sense of humour.

I remember our house was always busy with lots of company, entertainment, food and laughter. To prepare for the upcoming company, my mother would spend days in the kitchen, baking all kinds of fabulous

---

2 My father was diagnosed with prostate cancer one day before his 85th birthday, just 22 months after my own diagnosis. His Gleason score is 4 + 4 = 8 with a PSA of 13.5 ng/ml. The results of a bone and CT scan indicate no evidence cancer had spread outside the prostate. After speaking with a urologist, a radiation oncologist and the BC Cancer clinic, he's opted for active surveillance. If his PSA continues to rise, he may consider treatment.

3 Rosemary "Dolly" Gagnon (née McRobb) was born in Shaunavon, Saskatchewan, in 1934. Her mother, Annie Jane McRobb (née Reid), was from North Dakota, USA, and her father, David McRobb, emigrated to Canada from Aberdeen, Scotland.

goodies. Some of my favourites were lemon tarts, Nanaimo bars, cheesecake, chocolate cake, pinwheel cookies and of course, chocolate chip cookies. She would store Tupperware containers of treats in the freezer for our visitors to enjoy.

However, the snacks rarely lasted long enough for the next set of visitors. I used to raid the freezer at night and got used to eating frozen snacks, often consuming the entire contents of a container. I remember my mother yelling out my name in anger. "Gogs!"[4] she'd exclaim as she discovered the empty containers just before visitors arrived. Luckily for me, she'd always find something to serve.

Later in life, my mother and I often recalled fond memories of those days, and she continued to bake goodies for many years. Sadly, she passed away from congestive heart failure in 2015 at the age of 81. I miss her and her fabulous desserts.

That brings us back to the beginning of my story. The year was 2012. I was 52 years old, in good health and excellent physical condition — or so I thought.

---

4   Gogs is a childhood nickname given to me by my relatives, the McRobb family. We were next-door neighbours for over 15 years, and I grew up with my cousin Bruce. Unfortunately, he passed away in 2009 at the age of 50. To honour him and the family, I legally changed my name at that time.

CHAPTER TWO

ANNUAL CHECKUP

Lightning makes no sound until it strikes.

— Martin Luther King, Jr.

RISING PSA

THIS IS WHERE my prostate cancer story begins. I had started having annual checkups two years previous, at age fifty. These aren't really like a fitness challenge, where you lift weights, run on a treadmill and complete an obstacle course — although that sounds like fun. It's more general and tailored to your particular needs. The doctor will ask you several questions about your health, check your vital signs and address any of your concerns.

It was time again for my annual checkup. As expected, I passed with flying colours. Next, it was time to visit the lab for a few blood tests.

• • •

About a week later, I was back in the doctor's office to review the results. He seemed very pleased and commented that everything looked excellent, except that my PSA (prostate-specific antigen) was a bit higher than average, with a reading of 4.2 ng/ml (nanograms per millilitre). Despite having had two previous annual checkups, this was the first time my PSA had been tested. I didn't know much about it or what reading was deemed normal.

The doctor told me that the PSA is a measure of a protein that is produced by the prostate,[5] and testing it may help detect early prostate cancer. For men my age, ideal results are under 4.0. This was my first PSA test, and the results of 4.2 were only slightly higher than normal, so there was no cause for alarm.

He spoke of other reasons for an elevated PSA, such as an enlarged or inflamed prostate, or recent sexual activity. "Aha! That's probably it," I said, pointing to the doctor. He laughed and advised that it would be best to repeat the PSA blood test in three months.

That sounded great, and my mind was at ease

---

5   Located directly under the bladder, the prostate is a walnut-shaped gland responsible for making part of the fluid for semen. Its size varies with age.

knowing that PSA can vary for many reasons and one reading only slightly higher than normal was nothing to fret about. I felt good about the news. As I was about to leave, the doctor asked me to jump up onto the table for "a quick DRE."

"DRE?" I inquired.

"The digital rectal examination is no big deal," he replied. "I just check your prostate for any lumps or abnormalities, and it only takes a few moments."

"No problem," I said, and hopped up onto the table. He asked me to pull down my pants, roll over to my side facing the wall and to bend my knees up towards my chest. "Okay," I thought, "whatever you say, Doc."

He had put on gloves and spread some lubricant on his pointer finger. He said, "Just relax and breathe normally."

The examination only lasted about 15 to 20 seconds. Afterward, he said my prostate felt very smooth and normal, perhaps slightly enlarged, but not to lose sleep over it.

With that, I thanked him and got dressed. While leaving, my thoughts were on my prostate. Was it really slightly enlarged? Maybe it was average size for me? After all, I'm six feet two inches tall and weigh 200 pounds. Besides, doesn't everybody have different body sizes?

• • •

During the next three months, I never really thought about my PSA, prostate or health at all. I didn't talk about it with anybody, as it just wasn't on my mind. Furthermore, I felt fine and had tons of energy. It was really just business as usual, living my life, spending time with family and friends, hitting the gym, training in martial arts and riding my bike to and from my job as a computer programmer.

Before I knew it, the three months had flown by. I repeated the PSA blood test and returned to the doctor's office to review the results. This time, I fully expected the results to be under 4.0, as I'd held off on the sexual activity for a few weeks before the test.

Therefore, it was a shock when the doctor said the latest results were even higher than before, with a reading of 4.6. I couldn't believe it.

At first, I assumed the doctor would ask me to repeat the PSA blood test in another three months. Instead, he explained that although this was only the second PSA test in my entire life, he was troubled by the amount of the increase in such a short time. My PSA had increased by 0.4 in just three months. That didn't sound like much of an increase to me, but it was enough for him to recommend that I see a urologist.

This time, it was no surprise when he asked me to jump up onto the table for another quick you-know-what. (Actually, the doctor is right. The DRE is no big deal. Just relax, and it's over in no time.)

Again, he said my prostate felt very smooth and normal, except for being slightly enlarged. Okay, maybe my prostate was larger than in other men my age, but at least it was nice and smooth. I took that as a good sign.

While I was getting dressed, the doctor said to expect a call from the urologist. I thanked him, and he said not to worry. "What?" I thought. "Why would I be worried? My prostate's nice and smooth and probably normal for my size." I was a little disturbed by his tone, though, and wondered about the role of a urologist and why I must see one.

In retrospect, it's best to find ways to distract yourself from worry as it can lead to unnecessary stress and anxiety.

> I've suffered a great many catastrophes in my life. Most of them never happened.
>
> — Attributed to Mark Twain

The Urologist

As the days and weeks passed, I didn't think too much about my upcoming visit with the urologist and kept myself busy. I did do a little research on the subject and felt confident that there was nothing seriously wrong. Perhaps just an enlarged prostate, typical for aging men. It might not have anything to do with cancer.

Besides, I felt all right and didn't have any notable symptoms. I slept throughout the night without the need to use the washroom. I had no pain or discomfort. Everything was functioning 'down there' as expected and on command. Generally, I felt confident that there couldn't be anything seriously wrong. But once in a while I would wonder why my PSA was rising. Then I'd shake it off, reminding myself that my PSA results and prostate size were probably normal for me. After all, I'd only had a couple of readings, surely not enough for any conclusive results. That said, I was looking forward to my visit with the urologist to find out if anything was wrong.

• • •

So there I was at the urologist's office, filling out a form, answering general questions about my health. While pondering each question, I couldn't help but note I was the youngest one in the room. All the other men appeared to be in their seventies and eighties. They all seemed to be in good health, which caused me to wonder about the purpose of their visits.

Soon enough, my name was called. I handed in the completed form and was directed down a narrow hallway into a small room, invited to sit on a low stool and told that the urologist would see me soon.

While waiting, I started to think about the possibility of having cancer. That was a scary thought and one that got my heart pumping. It was comforting to know, however, that there was no history of prostate cancer in my family. I reminded myself again that I had only had two PSA tests and my prostate was nice and smooth. However, deep down, I knew that just about anything was possible, even if I didn't want to accept it as true.

Deep in thought, I was startled by the door as it opened. The urologist walked in, introduced himself and started to ask all kinds of questions about my health, especially regarding sexual health, ability to perform and my urination routine. Hearing the words 'perform' and 'routine' struck me as kind of funny — I pictured myself on stage, doing a song and dance show. I guess that was my way of lightening the mood.

I was happy to tell the urologist that I had no trouble 'performing,' at least in my opinion, and was able to sleep the night away without the need to get up and pee. He continued to ask questions, and I continued to answer with a perfect score of "No issues," except for just one thing.

It wasn't really a concern, and I wasn't even going to mention it, but thought it was essential to give full disclosure, as it was, after all, for my own health benefit.

The issue, which I didn't see as an issue, was that I had a bit of trouble using public urinals while other men are standing right beside me. I like some privacy, and if the washroom is empty, I tend not to have a problem. I figured I was just bladder-shy and pointed out that I could usually overcome this by focusing my mind on other things, like warm, sunny beaches and beautiful women.

After the urologist stopped laughing, he didn't seem too concerned and asked me to get up onto the table for an examination. I was getting quite used to this procedure and was more than happy to have a second opinion on my prostate.

I hopped up onto the table, pulled down my pants and assumed the position. I expected the examination to be the usual 15 to 20 seconds. However, it seemed to last much longer. The urologist took his time to feel everything within reach. After a while, it was a bit unpleasant, and I wondered if he had found a tumour.

When it was finally over, I was eager to hear about his findings. He reported that my prostate felt very smooth and normal, except for being slightly enlarged. Okay, I had to admit it: I had an enlarged prostate. However, the doctor said that it was possible that my PSA results were normal for me and not to worry about it.

Of course, I was quite happy and relieved, and I assumed that was the end of it. While I was getting dressed, the urologist recommended that I repeat the PSA blood test in six months and review the results with him then.

Knowing that the PSA is usually an annual test, I couldn't help but think that something might be wrong. The doctors kept telling me that everything was normal and not to be concerned, yet they also kept asking me to repeat the test.

Of course, I agreed. However, this time I decided it was time to share my PSA results with family and friends. And after scheduling my next appointment, I left the urologist's office on a mission: to do some serious research.

• • •

After the six months and the third PSA blood test, I was back at the urologist's office to review the results. However, this time, I was prepared. Since my last visit, I had changed my diet, eliminated junk food, trained longer at martial arts classes and worked out harder in the gym. As a result, I had lost 15 pounds and felt stronger than ever at 185 pounds.

This time, I was confident that my PSA results would be well below 4.0 and was expecting the doctor to congratulate me on the improvements.

Again, though, I was in for a shock. My PSA was still on the rise, and the latest results were 5.6. I was up a full point in the past six months and up 1.4 over the past nine months.

My heart sank. My head was filled with thoughts: "You mean I gave up all that junk food for nothing? Trained like a madman and pumped iron every day? All those delicious cookies and cakes I could have eaten . . ." The news was disappointing, and I felt like running to the bakery to drown my sorrows with a big piece of cake.

The urologist asked me to get up onto the table. Well, you know the drill. By this point, it was becoming entirely automatic for me to assume the position without question. As I expected (and appreciated), he took his time to do a thorough check. If there was anything to find, I certainly wanted him to find it.

After the examination was over, he said, "There's good news and bad news."

"Good grief," I mumbled, and asked for the good news first.

The good news was my prostate felt very smooth, and other than being slightly enlarged, it hadn't changed since my last visit. "What?" I thought. "All my efforts to improve my diet, exercise and lose weight had no effect on the size of my prostate?"

"Okay," I said, "what's the bad news?"

The bad news was the urologist was very concerned by the rapid rise in the PSA results. Even though my PSA was higher than average, he said, he wouldn't have been too bothered if it had stayed at the same level or had gone up just a little. However, my PSA had increased by 1.0 in only six months and he wasn't able to reach the entire prostate with a DRE. This hinted at the possibility there was a cancer tumour just out of reach.

He said, with a solemn tone, "I recommend a prostate biopsy."

My heart started to pound. I had become familiar with this procedure by doing research since my last visit. It sounded a bit like the alien anal probe I had heard about as a kid. Seeing an alien would be cool, but the probe was something you'd probably want to avoid.

During a prostate biopsy procedure, the doctor inserts an ultrasound probe into your rectum. Attached to the probe is a biopsy gun with a spring-driven hollow needle aimed at specific areas of the prostate. The biopsy gun shoots the needle (yes, by pulling a trigger) through the rectal wall into the prostate and retrieves tissue samples to be examined for cancer or other abnormalities in the pathology lab. The needle is shot through the rectal wall and into the prostate not once but multiple times at different locations.

After some thought, I realized I would perhaps prefer the alien anal probe. At least I'd get to see an alien.

The urologist continued to explain that the procedure involved potential risks, including bleeding at the biopsy site, blood in the semen, blood in the urine, difficulty urinating and infection. As a precautionary measure to help reduce the risk of an infection, he gave me a prescription for a three-day supply of antibiotics. I was instructed to take one pill twice a day, starting the day before the biopsy. That was two pills the day before the biopsy, two pills the day of the biopsy and two pills the day after the biopsy.

At this point, I was in a state of shock, and my head was spinning. None of this sounded any good.

Why wasn't there a less invasive test? Hadn't we made advancements in the medical field? I used to watch *Star Trek* as a kid. Where was the medical tricorder that could examine patients in an instant? I wanted to see Dr. Leonard H. "Bones" McCoy!

Unfortunately, the *Star Trek* technology doesn't exist, or at least it wasn't offered to me as an option.

Before the news of the rapid rise of my PSA, the DRE not being able to reach my entire prostate and the need for a prostate biopsy, I had been looking forward to seeing the urologist. This wasn't the news I had expected.

I took a few deep breaths and reminded myself that it was essential to know the facts and to face problems head-on. The facts would be critical for making decisions regarding my health, so doing research would empower me and give me peace of mind.

Thus, I left the urologist's office on a high note. "Bring it on!" I said.

Captain James T. Kirk: You suspect some danger?
Mr. Spock: Insufficient facts always invite danger, Captain.
Captain James T. Kirk: Well, I'd better get some facts.

— Dialogue from the TV series *Star Trek*, "Space Seed" episode, 1967

PROSTATE BIOPSY

A FEW MONTHS after my visit with the urologist, I was in the hospital wearing a gown, being escorted down a long hallway to the biopsy room by a very polite nurse. It felt surreal. I was reminded of the phrase 'dead man walking', due to my unknown future and the thought of the biopsy gun being inserted into my rectum, shooting needles into my prostate. But I knew this was an important test and was ready to get it done. In fact, not only ready: I was looking forward to getting the results.

As I followed the nurse, I observed other poor souls in hospital gowns with blank looks on their faces. I was determined not to look as glum as the other patients and decided to walk with my head held high and my chest out. I imagined inserting the biopsy gun and pressing the trigger myself with a smile. I told myself that this was going to be a piece of cake.

In the biopsy room, the nurse pointed to a table and asked me to lie down on my back. I was a bit confused, as I'd thought I should be on my side, in the same position as I assumed for a DRE. However, I complied. Soon, a doctor entered and picked up what looked like a garden hose. He introduced himself and revealed that I was about to have a bonus procedure, a cystoscopy, as a prelude to the main prostate biopsy event.

"So, what's up with the garden hose?" I asked, trying to sound casual.

He laughed and explained that it was a long thin tube with a light and a camera that would be inserted into my penis, down my urethra, through the prostate and into the bladder. This procedure allowed him to get a good look inside to check for abnormalities. The doctor applied some numbing jelly to my urethra and after a minute or so began the cystoscopy procedure.

"Are you sure that garden hose is going to fit?" I asked.

"Oh, yes, it will fit all right," he replied with a grin.

As it was going in, I used a mind trick I had learned back in 1985 — the early days of my martial arts training — to focus and quiet my mind, using the power of meditation to achieve inner calm. It was a bit tricky to concentrate, however, as I could feel the tube moving into my penis and down my urethra.

The doctor warned me before he pushed the tube into my bladder and I yelped a bit as it entered. Although it didn't hurt, it was a shocking, strange sensation — no doubt unlike anything I had experienced in the past.

Once the tube was inside, the doctor used the tube to inflate the bladder with a sterile solution. This would allow him to get a better look inside. As my bladder filled, he cautioned that I might feel the need to urinate, but not to hold back and to just let it go. That made me laugh out loud. I wasn't about to pee on the table and possibly on the doctor or myself. I just kept my mind focused, quiet and calm.

After a few minutes, the doctor said that it was time to remove the cystoscope. "Wiggle your toes and breathe deeply," he advised.

It took him only a few seconds to remove the entire tube. I felt relieved and pleasantly surprised that the procedure hadn't been as bad as I'd imagined. It seems your imagination can run wild in the face of the unknown. I needed to keep that in mind moving forward.

The first procedure was finished, and the doctor told me I could get up, use the washroom and prepare for the next one.

"That's right," I said. "That was just the preshow to the main event." The doctor chuckled.

In the washroom, I had a bit of trouble starting my flow of urine, partly due to my bladder shyness, but mostly because it burned a little to pee. However, the burning sensation lasted only a few seconds. The volume picked up and continued pain-free . . . for nearly a minute.

Wow, the doctor must have really filled up my bladder — this pee had to be a personal record! Nothing like the simple pleasures in life, I thought. It was an intense relief.

After washing my hands, I walked back to the table, where the nurse was waiting. This time, she asked me to lie down on my side and to bend my knees up towards my chest. This was the position that I had previously anticipated. It was time for the main event.

The nurse detailed what to expect, most of which I'd already learned from the urologist and my research. It was nice to hear it again, though, I thought, in case there was something I had forgotten or if there was any additional information.

Indeed, she had new information, and it was fairly significant.

"The biopsy gun makes a loud bang when it's fired, so don't be alarmed," she said.

The doctor entered the room, the same one who performed the cystoscopy. This time, he picked up what looked like a phaser from Star Trek. This turned out to be an ultrasound probe.

Malcolm Reed: They're called phase pistols. They have two settings, stun and kill. It would be best not to confuse them.

— Dialogue from the TV series *Enterprise*, "Broken Bow" episode, 2001

As the doctor gently inserted the ultrasound probe into my rectum and guided it towards my prostate, he said once it was in the right position, I would hear a loud bang and not to worry.

Bang!

Yikes! Despite the warning I still jumped. It was a lot louder than I'd expected, but I didn't feel a thing. No pain of any kind.

I wondered if the biopsy gun had misfired.

That was, until the second shot.

Bang!

Yow! That one felt like a bee sting deep inside my rectum. I yelled out and immediately felt embarrassed, as the pain had lasted only a few seconds. The nurse raised her eyebrows at me, and I said that I was all right.

"Unbelievable," I muttered to myself. On the pain scale, I'd gone from a level 10 to a level 0 in just a few seconds.

The doctor continued to reposition and fire the biopsy gun a total of six times, and then said, "All done. You can expect the results in about a week or so."

The whole thing had lasted only about 5 to 10 minutes. I was surprised it was over so quickly.

"That was it?" I said quietly, "That was no big deal."

It turned out that I didn't need Dr. Leonard H. "Bones" McCoy and his medical tricorder from *Star Trek* after all. Again, I reminded myself not to let my imagination run wild and to keep a level head.

Captain James T. Kirk: You know, the greatest danger facing us is ourselves, an irrational fear of the unknown. There's no such thing as the unknown, only things temporarily hidden, temporarily not understood.

— Dialogue from the TV series *Star Trek*, "The Corbomite Maneuver" episode, 1966

Later that evening, I discovered that the urologist was right about the risk of peeing blood. Although this is normal after a cystoscopy, it's a disturbing sight if you're not used to it. At first, it looked like something was seriously wrong, when in fact everything was just fine. Similar to what I'd felt earlier in the day, there was a burning sensation at the start, which lasted only a few seconds. I found that drinking lots of water helped to flush out my bladder and eliminate the burning feeling.

• • •

A week after the cystoscopy and prostate biopsy, I was back at the urologist's office to review the results.

The news was fantastic: no cancer found!

I was free to go, with the recommendation to get a PSA blood test once a year. If my results continued to rise, the testing frequency might increase to once every six or even three months, or I might be sent for another prostate biopsy.

It felt like I had just dodged a bullet — at least, at the time.

CHAPTER THREE

PROSTATE CANCER TESTING

Courage is being scared to death but saddling up anyway.

— John Wayne

If you want to conquer fear, don't sit home and think about it. Go out and get busy.

— Dale Carnegie

THE UROLOGIST ANEW

WE MOVED FROM Victoria to Vancouver Island's Comox Valley in 2015, which necessitated finding a new family doctor and urologist. Fortunately, we soon found terrific doctors and had all of our medical records forwarded to them.

Since the prostate biopsy in 2012, my PSA levels had continued to rise and were being monitored on a regular basis. By November 2016, I'd been taking a PSA blood test every three months for the past two years. Results fluctuated from 5.6 to a high of 7.8, with an upward trend.

Our new family doctor confirmed my prostate was nice and smooth, but she thought I should see the local urologist due to my continued rising PSA levels.

• • •

About a week later, my new urologist did a quick DRE. Since my PSA had been elevated for several years and had continued to rise, and my prostate biopsy of four years ago hadn't found any cancer, he recommended an MRI scan for three-dimensional imaging of my prostate. The idea was to use the results of the scan to identify any suspect areas of the prostate for targeting in "the next prostate biopsy."

"Say what, now?" I thought. "Another prostate biopsy?"

After a bit of hesitation, I agreed to go forward. The procedure was no big deal, and besides, who was afraid of that cap gun, anyway?

MRI Scan

The MRI scan (magnetic resonance imaging) was scheduled for the morning of December 5. No preparation was necessary, although Mary and I skipped breakfast and didn't drink anything. We hopped into the car, drove to the hospital and checked in at the medical imaging department.

In a private room, a nurse asked me to strip down, remove any jewellery, put on a hospital gown and have a seat in the hallway next to the exit door. Then I had to fill out a form with general questions about my health.

Since it was December, it was cold outside. I was also cold, because I was wearing only a thin hospital gown and sitting next to an exit door that kept opening. I realized it would soon be necessary to walk out to the mobile MRI unit parked outside.

"Oh well," I thought. "No big deal. So it's cold outside."

Soon, a nurse called my name, took my completed form and escorted me outside and onto a small lift on the side of the mobile MRI unit. As we rode the lift upwards, I waved to a few passers-by. Once the lift stopped, a large door opened and a very bright set of lights shone down on us as we walked inside. It brought to mind the possibility that a UFO had abducted me for the you-know-what. The inside appeared quite UFO-like, too — everything seemed futuristic, with a sterile feeling and advanced-looking gizmos and gadgets. One control panel was so appealing I wanted to examine it in more detail to see if I could fly this UFO out of here.

The nurse interrupted my thoughts and asked me to follow her through a door beside the control panel to the scanner room. The scanner was impressive, filling most of the room. A centre table attached to a very large tube resembled a sleeping chamber that might be used for long-term space travel. It inspired more thoughts of a possible UFO abduction.

The nurse cautioned that the scanner would make all kinds of loud noises and I would need to wear earplugs. She pointed to a table and asked me to lie down on my back. To help the scanner make clear images, she injected me with a special dye and instructed me to remain very still for the duration of the scan, about 45 minutes. I didn't feel the injection, as I was too focused on finding a comfortable position for the lengthy scan.

The nurse placed headphones over my earplugs[6] so we could hear each other during the scan. "Why would we need to hear each other?" I wondered. "Will I be *screaming* or something?"

She handed me a call bell that, if pressed, would immediately shut down the scan. I thanked her as she left the room and thought that since this was an important test, there was no way I was going to stop it.

Her voice came through on the headphones. "Can you hear me?" she asked.

"Yes, loud and clear," I replied. At that point, the table started to slide slowly into the giant tube. I began to realize that the tube was small on the inside and it was a good thing I'm not claustrophobic — it

---

6 Seemed counterproductive, but worked. Even though the earplugs muffled the scan noise, I was still able to hear through the headphones.

was a tight fit. Once my body was in the tube, the table stopped, leaving my head on the outside.

After a few moments of silence, I heard a different voice from the headphones, asking if I was ready for the scan.

I said, "No problem. Let's fire this thing up."

Instantly, the scanner came to life with loud banging and clanging noises that made it sound like it was breaking apart.

A voice on the headphones reminded me to stay still. I focused my mind on a warm, sunny beach and somehow found a rhythm in the random loud noises. After about half an hour, I couldn't tell if my arms were resting by my sides or floating in the air. I did my best not to move and figured that my arms must still be where they should be, since there had been no notification through the headphones.

After another 15 minutes or so, the scanner turned off, and a voice through the headphones said the scan was complete. "You did a great job."

That seemed a bit odd, as the scanner had done all the work while I'd remained still.

As the table slid out of the tube, the nurse removed the headphones and earplugs and said the results should be available in about a week or so. She escorted me down the lift and back into the hospital, where I got dressed.

I met Mary in the waiting area, and we went out for breakfast.

• • •

A few weeks later, on December 20, I was back at the urologist's office to get the results of the three-dimensional MRI scan.

The report was not good.[7]

There was an abnormal area of my prostate that was suspected to harbour high-grade prostate cancer. Located in an area that couldn't be examined by a DRE, this abnormality could account for my rising PSA.

It wasn't easy listening to the results, and I didn't like to hear the words 'abnormal' and 'suspect,' and especially not 'high-grade' and 'cancer.' But it was essential to remain calm and take the time to understand and process all of the information. After all, cancer was only *suspected*, not confirmed.

The urologist gave me a copy of the MRI scan report to review, and two statements immediately jumped out, so I asked him to elaborate.

The first statement — *Rectum is unremarkable* — initially seemed amusing. According to the urologist, it meant the rectum was either normal or had small abnormalities of no significance.

"Ah, okay," was what I said. What I thought was, "Is it a good idea to use a statement that has two different meanings? Is my rectum normal or not? Why not make this report easier to understand?"

---

7   The news put a damper on the holiday season, although we did our best to stay positive.

Anyway, I was more disturbed about the other statement.

The second statement was *Features are worrisome for a high-grade prostate malignancy.* There was nothing amusing about those words.

The urologist explained that the prostate has four zones. The largest is the peripheral zone, where most cancers are found, within reach of the DRE. The transition zone surrounds the urethra and grows larger as men age. The central zone usually doesn't have cancer, and the anterior zone is out of reach of the DRE, but only rarely has cancer.

In my case, the MRI indicated that the worrisome features were in the anterior zone of the prostate, an area that rarely has cancer.

"Of course," I said, "it would have to be in that zone."

This discovery shed light on why the results of my previous DREs and the prostate biopsy had reported everything to be normal. The anterior zone was out of reach of the DRE, and the biopsy may not have sampled this area due to the rare chance of its being cancerous.

After reviewing the MRI scan report with me, the urologist strongly encouraged me to go for another prostate biopsy, this time to target the anterior zone.

I paused and thought about my response. I was a bit scared, not of the prostate biopsy but of the potential results. I had to remind myself that I needed to find out if the MRI scan's results were indeed anything to worry about or not.

Therefore, "Bring it on, again!" I said.

Prostate Biopsy Reloaded

The second prostate biopsy was on February 28, 2017, and it was pretty much the same as the first, but without a cystoscopy.

Also, I didn't jump at the loud bangs this time.

As the doctor proceeded to insert the ultrasound probe, I imagined my body parts arguing over who had it worse.

Rectum: Looks like I'm a goner this time. There's a target on my head.

Penis: You only have to tolerate the ultrasound probe for a few minutes and take a couple of needles through the rectal wall. I'd take that any day over being violated by that garden hose.

Rectum: Garden hose? It's just a thin tube, and there's no pain. I'm the one who must suffer.

Penis: But your pain will go away in a few days. I must endure the awful memories. I will never get that image out of my head.

Rectum: I can see the biopsy gun, and it's getting closer. Tell the family I love them.

Prostate: You fellas are nuts! I'm the one they're gunning for, and I say bring it on!

Gogs: Okay, enough, boys. Just relax and breathe normally and we'll be out of here soon.

The best thing about this prostate biopsy was the absolute painlessness of the first four shots from the biopsy gun into my prostate. I didn't feel a thing. It was completely painless (except for the imaginary quarrel).

There were only two more shots to go. "This is a piece of cake," I thought.

The doctor must have known the fifth shot was going to hurt, because he mentioned, "This one might hurt a bit," as he pulled the trigger.

Bang!

I yelled out in pain. This shot felt like a *hornet* sting deep inside my rectum, rather than a mere bee sting, and the pain lasted much longer than a few seconds. He apologized and said there was just one more to go. Then he fired for the sixth and final time.

It was a relief to have made it through another prostate biopsy. The doctor said to expect the results in about a week or so and wished me luck.

"Why is he wishing me luck?" I pondered. That didn't sound too reassuring, nor did the way he said it. I took it as a clue — he might have seen something abnormal, or perhaps knew something was wrong.

I thanked him, got up from the table and walked to the washroom to clean up and get dressed. While walking, I experienced much more pain and discomfort than after the prostate biopsy four years ago. Though the pain wasn't unbearable, I felt noticeably more tender. On the pain scale, it was a level 6, compared to the level 2 I had experienced in the previous biopsy.

While getting dressed, my mind returned to the MRI scan results, most notably the statement *Features are worrisome for a high-grade prostate malignancy.*

I thought about how the urologist talked about abnormalities found in the anterior zone, where it's rare to find cancer and is out of reach of the DRE.

I thought about that fifth needle shot and the doctor's warning, and the sympathetic tone of his voice when he wished me luck.

I thought maybe this prostate biopsy had been more painful because it was the first time the needle had hit this area. The previous urologist did say the first biopsy had no specific targets — the examined tissue samples were from areas where cancer was most likely to be found.

At the time, I didn't realize it was possible to have cancer when a biopsy was negative. But after all, the pathologist only examines the tissue samples, not the entire prostate.

It was reassuring to know, however, that the recent prostate biopsy had specific targets based on the results of the MRI scan. The fact that it was more painful was probably a good sign.

Once again, if there was cancer somewhere in my prostate, I certainly wanted the doctor to find it.

After getting dressed, I met Mary in the waiting area, and we walked out to the car, holding hands. After opening the passenger door, I was surprised to find a pillow and a note. The extra support was unexpected and appreciated.

I sat down in style. "Ah, nice and comfy," I said.

We've been married since 1982, and she's extremely loving and caring, always thinking about me. I felt blessed to have such a thoughtful and awesome wife in my life.

Oh yes, the note was private.

• • •

When we got home, our two dogs greeted us as if we were royalty. (It never ceases to amaze us how happy they are to see us every time we come home. It's almost like we've been away on a trip for weeks or months.)

I got down on my knees to greet them as usual, and both dogs gave a soft whimper. I knew they'd sensed I was troubled and in a bit of pain. They continued with a few more whimpers until I reassured them everything was fine.

I took some time to reflect on my good fortune in having a wonderful family with such caring pets. Both dogs were rescued from the shelter. Maya is a St. Bernard/German shepherd mix who weighs 110 pounds. She's been in our family for 10 years. We've had Nelly — an 80-pound German shepherd/border collie cross — in our family for nine years.

For the next week, Maya and Nelly followed me everywhere, stayed at my side, slept by my feet and looked up every so often to check on me. They provided tremendous companionship while Mary and I waited for the results of the second prostate biopsy.

• • •

About a week later, I was back at the urologist's office to review the results, and the report wasn't good.

He got right to the point. There was cancer in five of six tissue samples. Overall, 50 percent of the submitted tissue contained cancer.

He went on to tell me that I had a Gleason score of 7.[8] The Gleason score indicates how cancer cells look and act compared to healthy cells. It measures the cancer's growth rate and how likely it is to spread. The lower the score, the better.

To calculate the score, the pathologist examines the tissue samples and determines where cancer is most prominent and where it's next-most prominent, assigning a grade from 1 to 5 to each of these areas. My grade was 4/5 for the most prominent area and 3/5 for the next-most prominent area. This gave me a Gleason score of 4 + 3 = 7, indicating a high–intermediate risk for cancer that was growing at a moderate pace and usually needs treatment.

---

8   Two different Gleason scores add up to 7, either 3 + 4 or 4 + 3, and it's important to know how your score was determined. A score of 3 + 4 = 7 indicates a low–intermediate risk for cancer that's growing very slowly and sometimes doesn't need treatment. By contrast, a score of 4 + 3 = 7 indicates a high–intermediate risk for cancer that's growing at a moderate pace and usually requires treatment.

My first thought was "I'm going to die."

I started to feel sick and weak. My vision blurred and my mind turned into a hazy fog. The sound of my pounding heartbeat drowned out the urologist's voice. I blanked out for a few seconds or so, trying to process the fact that I had prostate cancer.

The fact it was growing at a moderate pace had me worried. My thoughts turned to the most important things in life: my family, how they'd manage, how much I'd miss being in their lives, our dogs, and all the things I still wanted to achieve. I had flashbacks of past memorable moments and I thought about how much life was worth living. I wasn't ready for death.

Commander Spock: Fear of death is illogical.
Dr. Leonard H. "Bones" McCoy: Fear of death is what keeps us alive.

— Dialogue from the movie *Star Trek: Beyond*, 2016

Please note this is a typical reaction and most men will experience similar feelings when diagnosed with cancer. However, hindsight shows this was an overreaction, as I hadn't yet learned all the facts. It's easy to jump to conclusions and react on insufficient information. We need to refrain from thinking cancer is synonymous with death. It's important to stay calm and allow yourself time to process and understand the situation.

At the time, I didn't realize it was possible to ask for a second opinion on the Gleason score. Since it requires human evaluation under a microscope, it's possible to make a mistake. Perhaps the results are lower or even higher than reported, which may influence the treatment decision. Evaluating prostate biopsies is challenging and requires an experienced pathologist. In my case, it turns out the pathologist was very experienced, although it would have been nice to know that fact at the time.

Out of nowhere, a voice in my head said: "You're not dead yet." Exactly the words I needed to hear! I realized that I was very much alive and had a crucial role to play in my future.

I repeated the words: "You're not dead yet!"

Snapping out of the hazy fog, I bombarded the urologist with questions. "Do I need immediate treatment? Has the cancer spread? What's the risk of doing nothing? How much time do I have? What are my options? Are there other tests to help decide on treatment? If I choose surgery, what are the side effects? What about sexual function and urinary incontinence? Can permanent side effects be treated? How long have you been a surgeon? How many men have you treated? How many suffer from permanent side effects? How many men similar to my age and condition have fully recovered? How long is the recovery process? What's the risk of recurrence compared to other treatments? Do I need to prepare for surgery? How do you do the surgery? Can we improve the chances to minimize side effects? What happens if surgery fails to remove all cancer? What do you do with my prostate after it's cut out?"

In retrospect, I realize my questions were mostly surgery-focused, when it would have been best to ask more about other treatment options. In the back of my mind, I was already leaning towards surgery. However, it's essential to keep an open mind to explore other possibilities, and I shouldn't have made a snap judgement without all the facts. Ideally, decisions should be based on logic, not necessarily emotion. You can always ask similar questions of your health-care team[9] and replace the word 'surgery' with another treatment option.

Throughout the questioning, the urologist was very patient and calm, demonstrating real compassion, and it became evident that he sincerely cared about me. His knowledge was remarkable, and he took his time to answer all my questions. I'm sure that if I'd had a hundred more, he would've happily answered them all. Not only was he compassionate, but he also displayed a great passion for his job — something that we had in common.

The good news was that the prostate biopsy results indicated the cancer hadn't spread outside of the prostate. To be certain, the urologist suggested a few

---

9   Your health-care team is an individual choice made up of members you trust and not limited to medical doctors, urologists, radiation oncologists, medical oncologists, nutritionists, physical rehabilitation, emotional, and spiritual support therapists.

additional tests, including a bone scan and a CT scan. I was fully cooperative and agreed to further testing.

He provided a mountain of reading material and discussed potential treatment options, including chemotherapy, radiation and radical prostatectomy surgery. Each treatment has the goal of destroying cancer cells — chemotherapy uses drugs, radiation uses high-energy rays or particles and surgery aims to remove the cancer.

For each option, there were many different techniques,[10] so he referred me to the reading material for more details. Whichever route I chose, I would have to undergo lifetime follow-up monitoring to ensure the cancer didn't return.

The urologist described in detail the potential risks and side effects of each treatment. The two side effects common to each treatment that scared me the most were urinary incontinence and erectile dysfunction, with the possibility of being permanent.

It's important to discuss all the options with your health-care team, as the degree of risk of each side effect may vary with the treatment you choose. For example, one treatment may impose a higher risk for erectile dysfunction than another, even though the possibility exists for either option.

We discussed holding off on treatment and doing more PSA tests and prostate biopsies to monitor

---

10   Within each option, there are lots of possibilities for treatment. For example, there are different types of surgery, many forms of radiation and a variety of chemotherapy drugs.

cancer growth. This process is known as 'active surveillance.' But I eliminated that option — I wasn't keen on giving the cancer more time to grow and spread.

We knew cancer existed in five of six tissue samples, and the Gleason score of 4 + 3 = 7 indicated it was growing at a moderate pace and hadn't yet spread outside the prostate. Also, taking into account that 50 percent of the submitted tissue contained cancer, I wanted to deal with this right away. I was leaning towards surgery.

A radical prostatectomy is a surgical procedure that can be approached in four different ways. In the retropubic approach, the prostate is removed through an incision in the lower abdomen. A perineal procedure is done through an incision between the scrotum and anus. In the laparoscopic approach, the surgeon uses several small incisions and tube-like instruments to remove the prostate, while the robotic approach uses small incisions and remote-controlled robotic arms.

The urologist clarified that the laparoscopic and robotic approaches have potentially faster recovery times, less blood loss and less pain. However, these were not available at the local hospital. Between the two remaining approaches, the perineal is potentially a quicker procedure than the retropubic surgery. However, it has a higher risk of causing erectile dysfunction. Preserving erections was definitely a priority for us, therefore the retropubic approach would be the better choice if I opted for surgery at this hospital.

I asked him about his experience, and he described how many surgeries he'd performed, how many patients had required follow-up treatment and how many suffered from permanent side effects.

Mary and I both felt at ease with his calm nature, extensive knowledge and expertise in oncology surgery. (Not just a surgeon, he's also a clinical instructor at UBC in Vancouver, involved in teaching urology and family medicine residents as well as medical students. This makes it essential for him to keep up with the latest surgical techniques and other treatment options.)

We also felt confident in the retropubic approach and didn't deem it necessary to travel to another hospital, look for another surgeon who might perform one of the other radical prostatectomy methods, or even research different treatment options.

In retrospect I realize that even though my urologist discussed various treatment options, he didn't provide an exhaustive list. His knowledge — while extensive — is limited to his expertise and experience. It's imperative to give yourself the opportunity to talk with other doctors who are experts in other treatments. Even if surgery was the best option for me, I could have benefited from visiting BC Cancer and the Island Prostate Centre, both located in Victoria, and contacting the Vancouver Prostate Centre for more information and the opportunity to see other doctors.

The urologist encouraged us to take our time with the decision. He advised we speak with family and friends and suggested I make an appointment with a radiation oncologist, and possibly a medical oncologist, to learn about all my options.

Since I was leaning towards surgery and assumed there would be long wait times, I figured it'd be good to get on the list right away. I could always change the arrangements later, so I asked him to put me on his surgical waiting list for an open radical retropubic prostatectomy (an incision in the lower abdomen with an attempt to preserve erections).

Before we left, he encouraged us to call any time with any questions about treatment options and reminded me that I could make changes up to the day of surgery. We thanked him, shook his hand and felt good about our visit.

We left the office holding hands, and again I was on a mission to research and study the various treatment options.

In retrospect, even though reading and re-searching on my own provided useful information, it isolated Mary from the process. I spent many hours on the computer while she waited patiently in the wings. Ideally, this time should have been spent together, working and learning as a team.

I encourage you to be open and share your feelings and time with your partner and loved ones. Please don't feel the need to shelter them from the burden. Just like you, they, too, may feel helpless, scared and alone. This time together is an opportunity to strengthen your relationship, think more clearly and make sounder decisions.

During the drive home, I started to look over the stack of reading material and imagined another conversation among my body parts.

Prostate: Hey fellas, did you hear that? It looks like I'm not the one they're gunning for after all. There's cancer inside me, and they want to get rid of it.

Penis: That's good news, right, Prostate? Once they get rid of that cancer, you'll be okay, right?

Rectum: Uh, Penis, it doesn't really work that way.

Prostate: That's right, Rectum. To get rid of my cancer, they must get rid of me.

Penis: What? Isn't there another way?

Gogs: Hold on, boys, you're getting ahead of yourselves. We need a few more tests to see where we stand. And there's a lot of reading material to get through and research to do, and I need to talk with family and friends. Quite simply, we need more time to fully consider everything before making a decision.

Bone Scan

The bone scan was scheduled for March 21. No advance preparation was necessary. Its purpose was to see if any of the prostate cancer had spread from the prostate into my bones. (For some reason, prostate cancer has a very strong preference for bones.)

Mary and I arrived at the hospital and checked in at the medical imaging department. A nurse asked me to fill out a form with general questions about my health. By now, I'd filled out so many of these forms, I had all of the questions and answers memorized.

Another nurse soon called my name and took the completed form. He escorted me into a small room, asked me to take a seat and closed the door. He said that I'd be injected with a low dose of a radioactive substance called a tracer. The tracer would travel through my bloodstream and absorb into my bones. This would help the scanner detect any bone damage due to cancer, infections or other causes.

I watched him prepare the needle and fill it with the tracer. He noticed that I was a bit nervous and to lighten the mood he pretended to have a twitch in his hand while he attempted to get a proper grip on the needle. He said that this was the first time he'd ever used a needle — he hoped I didn't mind. He held his twitching hand with his other hand in efforts to control the needle as he pointed it towards my arm. It was evident that he was a seasoned professional and I had to laugh at the expression on his face. His performance calmed me down and helped to take my mind off the cancer.

As he injected me, I could feel the radioactive substance flowing through my veins. I was thinking how cool it would be if the injection gave me superpowers like *Spider-Man*. But, unfortunately, it didn't. After the injection, the nurse said that the tracer required about two hours to be absorbed into my bones before the scan. He asked me to drink at least three to four large glasses of water in the meantime. I thanked him and promised to return in about two hours.

While walking to the waiting area, I spotted a hydration station with a sign that reminded people to drink water before their bone scan. I was happy to see the station and filled up a couple of plastic glasses with water, then proceeded to the waiting area to rejoin my lovely wife. We held hands, and it was good to be together and just to sit back and breathe. Every once in a while, she'd remind me to drink the water, making sure I drank every drop.

As we waited and looked through magazines, Mary's phone rang. It was our daughter, Stacey. She said the hospital had called. My surgery was scheduled for May 1, and I needed to call back to schedule an appointment with the pre-admission nurse.

"No way!" I said. "I have a surgery date already?" Incredible — surgery in less than six weeks! I hadn't expected this to happen so soon.

I later learned that hospitals schedule surgeries based on patient wait time, urgency and availability of operating rooms, rather than queue order.

I hung up the phone before I thought to get the hospital's phone number from Stacey, so I walked to the administration desk to make the appointment.

At the administration desk, I explained my situation and asked to schedule an appointment with the pre-admission nurse. I was a bit shocked at the response from the lady at the desk: "You'll have to call the hospital to make an appointment."

I was already in the hospital, standing right in front of administrative staff. Yet I must phone the hospital to make an appointment? At a loss for words, I just walked away, confused.

On the way back to the waiting area, I stopped and repeated my request to the lady at the medical imaging desk. Her reply was a bit different: "You'll need to ask at the administration desk."

I wondered if this was some kind of an Abbott and Costello routine or if *Just for Laughs* was secretly filming.

"But the lady at the administration desk just told me I had to phone the hospital!" I said.

To my relief, the medical imaging receptionist replied, "Really? Okay, don't worry. I'll phone for you." She dialed a number on her desk phone and handed it to me.

After a few rings, the pre-admission nurse answered the phone. I was so excited that I messed up my words and wasn't making any sense. Once she understood who I was, she said, "Gogs! I see you're calling from within the hospital. Wait for me in the medical-imaging waiting area, and I'll be right down to see you!"

Her enthusiasm was encouraging, but I started to feel overwhelmed. Everything seemed to be moving too fast to process. I paused for a few seconds before replying with a simple "Okay."

I hung up the phone, thanked the lady at the desk and walked back to the waiting area while trying to gather my thoughts.

The friendly pre-admission nurse appeared within a few minutes. She was full of energy and seemed pleased to meet me. She confirmed that my surgery was scheduled for May 1 and I'd be first on the table at 8:15 a.m. As a bonus, I'd have two surgeons working as a team. I asked about cancellation if I decided on a different treatment option and she replied, "No problem, Gogs. If you have any doubts or need any more time, please feel free to cancel."

She handed me the surgery instructions, and we began to review the process. After some discussion, she registered the blank expression on my face and said, "You look like a deer caught in the headlights. Let me just leave you with the information." On a sticky note, she wrote my surgery date, her phone number and an appointment date of April 3 for a pre-admission checkup and visit with the anaesthesiologist. She put the sticky note on the surgery instructions and added, "Gogs, please call me if you have any questions." I nodded my head in agreement. As she walked away, she looked back and smiled, so I waved.

I couldn't help thinking, "What just happened?" While it was good to be on the list, I hadn't been expecting the surgery so quickly. My arms had goosebumps, and my heart started pounding. At this point, I began to second-guess myself and wondered if I was doing the right thing. Maybe this was moving way too fast.

While lost in thought, I was jolted back to reality by a different nurse calling my name. The two hours had passed quickly, and it was time for the bone scan. I was like a robot responding to the basic instructions: "Empty-bladder. Remove-jewellery. Strip. Put-on-gown. Follow-me." It all happened without thought, reminding me of the Star Trek Borg phrase "Resistance is futile."

The nurse directed me to lie on the scanner table under a huge camera. She asked me to remain very still for about an hour while the scan was in progress. That sounded very inviting. My mind was muddled and I needed a good lie-down. While I rested, the bone scanner fired up, and I remained still and tried not to think about anything. There was just too much to process and my brain needed time to reboot. I took solace in being under the giant camera, which was like a protective shield. I didn't want the scan to end.

About an hour later, though, the procedure was complete. I stood up, feeling vulnerable leaving the perceived safety of the scanner. After getting dressed, I rushed to see Mary, who greeted me with open arms. We walked to the car, holding on to each other, but my brain remained cloudy with disbelief about the rapid developments.

On the drive home, I stared out the window and thought about the importance of enjoying every moment in life. I looked over at Mary with tenderness and beamed.

Captain Jean-Luc Picard: Live now. Make now always the most precious time. Now will never come again.

— Dialogue from the TV series *Star Trek: The Next Generation*, "The Inner Light" episode, 1992

CT Scan

The CT (computed tomography) scan was set for the morning of March 24. Mary and I skipped breakfast, and we didn't drink anything. Although I had to fast, she didn't, but she was in this with me, physically and emotionally. She, too, was experiencing the pain and disbelief of my prostate cancer diagnosis. We truly were in this process together all the way.

The purpose of the CT scan was to see if any of the prostate cancer had spread beyond the prostate and into nearby lymph nodes and other organs or structures in my pelvis.

A nurse asked me to fill out a form and drink a glass of water. Once I'd done that, another nurse called my name, and it was time for the scan. It wasn't necessary to change into a hospital gown this time, but I did have to remove my belt. The nurse walked towards the scanner table and asked me to lie down on my back. She injected me intravenously with a substance to help the scanner make clearer images. With all of the needles I'd had up to this point, one more didn't even faze me.

During the injection, I felt a warming sensation, and the nurse suggested I might also sense a metallic taste in my mouth and feel the need to urinate.

"Not to worry," she added. "It's normal and should dissipate quickly."

Suddenly, it felt like I had just peed my pants. The nurse assured me that it was most likely the effects of the contrast substance. I hoped she was right, as she was about the metallic taste — yuck!

While waiting for the CT scanner to fire up, I studied its design. It looked like a big doughnut, a bit similar to the MRI scanner but without the long tube.

The nurse informed me that the scan was about to start, and told me to remain very still and that it might be necessary to hold my breath a few times during the procedure. I replied, "No problem. Let's fire this thing up."

The table began sliding in and out of the doughnut part of the scanner, and I wasn't sure what to expect next. It was surprisingly quiet, unlike the MRI scan. It made only slight buzzing, clicking and whirring sounds.

The scan was complete within about 30 minutes. I grabbed my belt, thanked the nurse, met Mary in the waiting area, and off we went to get something to eat. Our time together during this whole experience was becoming somewhat routine, but it further cemented our relationship.

And, oh yes, the nurse was right. My pants were dry.

THE DECISION

IT WAS MARCH 27, 2017. All the tests were complete and the results available. During the past few weeks, I had researched and read about various prostate cancer treatments, including options not available in Canada. I had talked with family, friends, neighbours and our family doctor. I had also spoken with a few prostate cancer survivors and listened to their stories.

One of the cancer survivors I spoke with had opted for seed implants, a form of internal radiation therapy known as brachytherapy. I first learned about him from my aunt who lives in Vancouver. She said that his treatment had been a few years ago and he was now doing just fine. For this procedure, low-dose radioactive seeds — each about the size of a grain of rice — are implanted into the prostate. The goal is to place the seeds close to the cancer cells to minimize damage to nearby healthy tissue. The seeds remain in the body permanently, but are only radioactive for a few months.

Being curious, I contacted him to listen to his story. It turned out that he was 81 years old when diagnosed with a Gleason score of 3 + 3 = 6, indicating a cancer that is growing very slowly and often doesn't require treatment.

After mulling over his options, he'd decided on low-dose seed implants, as he didn't like the idea of active surveillance or surgery. Since the procedure, his PSA had dropped to a low of 1.2 from 9.1 ng/ml. (After radiation, it's normal for PSA to rise and fall over the next two years. After that, if PSA rises by 2.0 or more above the lowest reading and continues to rise, it could be a sign the cancer is returning, and you may need to explore further treatment options.)

As far as side effects, he said everything was working as before, and he was happy. When I asked him about sex, he replied, "Listen, just because I'm an old man doesn't mean I want relations with an old lady, and at my age, I don't see any young women lined up at the door. So I play cards now." He was quite the character, full of wit and energy, and it was a pleasure to hear his story.

On recalling this conversation, I believe I missed out on the opportunity to connect with more cancer survivors before making my decision, especially men who were closer to my age when they were diagnosed. Just as important, I should have spoken with a radiation oncologist and possibly a medical oncologist to discuss more options, as my urologist suggested I do.

• • •

It was time for the appointment with the urologist. Mary and I were eagerly attentive as he summarized the test results and reviewed our options to help us decide on treatment.

The urologist's reality check began with my current PSA results, which were 7.8 ng/ml. During the past five years, my PSA had been tested fourteen times. When plotted on a chart, it revealed a disturbing upward trend, rising on average 0.72 per year.

He reminded us of the MRI that indicated a high-grade prostate malignancy in the anterior zone of the prostate, where cancer is rarely found, out of reach of a DRE.

He reviewed the results from the prostate biopsy: cancer in five of six tissue samples and a Gleason score of 4 + 3 = 7, indicating a high–intermediate risk for cancer growing at a moderate pace. Overall, 50 percent of the submitted tissue contained cancer.

He said the bone scan results showed no scintigraphic evidence of osseous metastatic disease — that is, there was no sign cancer had spread to my bones. There was, however, arthritis found in my left AC joint at the top of the shoulder. That made total sense, as about 20 years before, during shoulder roll practice in martial arts, I had had a terrible landing directly on my left shoulder. I didn't bother to have it checked out at the time and let it heal on its own. That decision turned out to be a bad one, as I've had chronic shoulder pain ever since. Let it serve as a reminder to you to always get proper medical care.

The urologist concluded by reviewing the CT scan, which had found no evidence of metastatic disease in the abdomen or pelvis, meaning no sign that cancer had spread outside of the prostate and into nearby lymph nodes and other organs or structures in my pelvis.

He did say there was a trace of plaque found in my aorta, the main artery in the body — no doubt a consequence of having eaten junk food for the past fifty years. Up to this point in my life, I've somehow managed to avoid high blood pressure and diabetes. However, I fully realize my eating habits must improve substantially. Otherwise, those ticking time bombs could explode.

After reviewing all of the test results, it was time for a final decision on treatment. The cancer was growing at a moderate pace and appeared to be confined within the prostate. At 57, I could expect to live many more years, increasing the risk the cancer would spread beyond the prostate. I felt healthy and strong enough to endure the surgery and recovery. I had fantastic support from the medical community and family. Also, if the operation somehow missed some of the cancer, there would be radiation, chemotherapy and other treatment options available.

For some reason, I wasn't too bothered about dealing with the potential side effects. My priority was to remove my prostate as fast as possible.

The urologist listed the three priorities of surgery in descending order of importance. One:

remove all cancer. Two: preserve urinary control. And three: maintain sexual function. Both sexual and urinary functions might be sacrificed if necessary to get all the cancer out. The fact that I was young and healthy hinted that I might have a better chance to overcome these side effects. But they could be permanent.

In that case, he pointed out, there are post-surgical medical treatments that may help resolve urinary incontinence and erectile dysfunction.

After careful deliberation and review of all the relevant factors, I opted for surgery. The urologist confirmed my appointment with the pre-admission nurse and the anaesthesiologist for the following week, on April 3, and my surgery date on May 1. We thanked him and shook his hand. On the way out, I thought of Jean-Luc Picard from *Star Trek: The Next Generation* and his catchphrase, "Make it so."

It's important for readers to understand that I'm not advocating one form of treatment over another. No single option is best for everyone. All options can be viable, depending on the different circumstances of each individual. While one treatment option may work for one individual, it may not work for another. Each case must be evaluated based on its own factors, such as test results, age, general health, life expectancy, personal preferences, prostate size[11] and available treatment

---

11   For larger prostates, your health-care team may examine ways to shrink or reduce the size, depending on your treatment choice. For example, brachytherapy may require a smaller prostate for more optimal treatment.

options. In some cases, more than one treatment may be required.

Mary and I left the office in high spirits, feeling confident about our decision. On the drive home, I imagined a slightly less spirited conversation among my body parts about the decision to proceed with surgery.

Penis: "Did I hear correctly? Are we going through with the surgery? Will Prostate die in five weeks?"

Rectum: "I'm afraid so, Penis. Life's not going to be the same without Prostate. It's a sad day for us."

Prostate: "Hey, fellas, I want you to know that I'm not dead yet! Cheer up! Let's make the best of it, and besides, don't I get a last request?"

Rectum: "Why sure, anything, Prostate, just name it."

Penis: "We can organize a party and invite a few close friends."

Rectum: "Of course, Penis, great idea."

Prostate: "Now you're talking my language. Best to enjoy life while still alive!"

Chapter Four

Pre-admission Testing

> If it can be solved, there's no need to worry, and if it
> can't be solved, worry is of no use.
>
> — The Dalai Lama

Pre-admission Nurse

After I made the decision to have surgery, I began a journal documenting my prostate cancer experience. I wrote about the various doctor's appointments, tests and results, and my thoughts and feelings at the time. Writing notes can be quite therapeutic, serving as a distraction to worry. This note-taking kept me busy and allowed me to process more information and reflect on the different experiences.

Ideally, I should have started journaling much sooner, as it would have given me more opportunity to contemplate my options.

On April 3, Mary and I checked in at the hospital administration desk at 8:30 a.m., well before our 9:00 a.m. appointment with the pre-admission nurse and the anesthesiologist. In the waiting area, we flipped through magazines and reassured each other that everything was going to be okay.

A few moments later, we saw the pre-admission nurse walking towards us with a big smile. She waved and called out, "Hello, Gogs," and asked us to follow her down a long hallway. After a few turns, she pointed to a door and said, "Here we are, my office."

After ushering us in, she closed the door and sat behind the desk. She confirmed my name, birthdate and other personal data. She proceeded to ask dozens of questions more detailed than in the standard forms. It made me realize how the urologist must have felt when I peppered him with questions.

She wanted to know everything about my physical health, sexual health and mental health; a complete history of previous operations, broken bones and illnesses; any medical concerns (other than the prostate cancer), a list of daily medications, supplements and vitamins; and family medical history. I didn't know all of the answers to her extensive questions, especially regarding family medical history, but I responded to the best of my knowledge.

It's important to be aware of your family medical history. I've since questioned my living relatives and encourage you to do the same.

Reliving my medical history reminded me of an experience from 1972. My cousin Bruce and I were 11 years old, taking delight in a full day by ourselves at the PNE (Pacific National Exhibition) in Vancouver. We were riding the Zipper when suddenly I felt a pain in my right side. The pain was so intense that I started to scream, which of course failed to attract attention, as every other kid on the ride was also screaming. It turned out that my appendix had ruptured. I ended up being hospitalized for two months and underwent three separate operations. The doctors reported that I came within an hour or so of final curtains.

Later that year, Bruce and I, along with a good buddy, went on a school ski trip to Mount Seymour in North Vancouver. We decided against ski lessons and took off on our own to the more advanced hills, where I broke my left leg in three places. I had to wear a cast for six months. I'll never forget the emergency room doctor asking my father to hold me down while he set my leg back into place. That was a real-life example of short-term pain for long-term gain. Although 1972 was a bad year health-wise, the year was full of fond memories of care and love from doctors, nurses, family and friends.

After an hour or so of questioning, the nurse recorded my blood pressure, weight and height and listened to my heart. The whole experience was very sobering and reminded me not to take health for granted. We've all heard that cliché before, but I was finally getting the message, perhaps realizing it might be possible to give up junk food without losing fond memories of childhood.

The pre-admission nurse concluded, "Okay, Gogs, we're all done here." She added that I still needed some blood work, an echocardiogram, an X-ray and a visit with the anesthesiologist.

She wrote this all down, with instructions on how to find each department, then handed me the stack of forms and pre-printed labels to hand out at each stop. With the stack of forms and labels in hand, we proceeded to our first destination, the blood-work lab.

The Laboratory

The lab was easy to find, since it was just down the hallway from the pre-admission nurse's office. I checked in at the desk, handed in the appropriate papers and labels and sat in the waiting area. The queue had only a few people, and the wait was only twenty minutes.

I followed the nurse to the lab and watched her reviewing my paperwork and labels. She confirmed my name and birthdate and put the pre-printed labels onto several small vials used to collect blood. I've had many blood tests in the past, and usually only two to three vials were required. This time there were twelve.

I thought, "Oh well, no big deal. How much blood can those small vials hold, anyway?" It was encouraging to know they'd be analyzed and would provide critical information to the surgical team.

The nurse proceeded to draw blood until all the vials were full. It was time to go. I looked at the instructions for the next stop, picked up Mary in the waiting area and off we went to the echocardiogram department.

ECHOCARDIOGRAM

LOCATING THE ECHOCARDIOGRAM DEPARTMENT wasn't straightforward. Trying to find it was a bit like a treasure hunt — without the thrill of finding the treasure. The hospital layout was fairly new to us, and we were lost despite the directions from the pre-admission nurse. I accepted the blame, as I'd insisted we could find the place without asking for help. Mary disagreed and wondered why we couldn't just take two seconds to ask for directions. She patiently followed me around the hospital, down long hallways, through doorways and up and down the elevator.

> Captain James Kirk: Our species can only survive if we have obstacles to overcome. You remove those obstacles. Without them to strengthen us, we will weaken and die.
>
> — Dialogue from the TV series *Star Trek*, "Metamorphosis" episode, 1967

After 15 minutes of getting nowhere, Mary asked a passing nurse for directions. It turned out that we had walked by the echocardiogram department a few times. Mary was right — I must learn to ask for directions.

We checked in, and the lady at the desk said, "You've arrived at a good time. You just missed a big lineup."

I looked at Mary and said, "Good thing we got lost." The look on her face told me that keeping my mouth shut would have been a wiser choice. (Although she apologized later and kissed me on the neck.)

After check-in, a nurse escorted me into a small room and asked me to remove my shirt and lie down on the table. There would be two different procedures in this department: an electrocardiogram and an echocardiogram.

For the electrocardiogram, the nurse attached about a dozen electrodes to various locations around my chest. After connecting the wires to a machine, she turned it on, and the device began to print out. It reminded me of a stock ticker machine: the paper rolled out of the back while a needle moved back and forth, recording the rhythm of my heartbeat.

After a few minutes, the nurse turned off the machine and removed the electrodes. She tore off the paper from the back of the device, held it up to see the results and announced it was time for the next procedure.

For the echocardiogram, the nurse turned down the lights, then applied gel to an ultrasound probe and rubbed it on my chest. She moved the probe back and forth as black and white images of my heart appeared on the computer screen that sat on the table beside me. Every so often, she'd ask me to hold my breath as she continued moving the probe.

The procedure was completed in about 20 minutes. The nurse wiped the gel off my chest, and after I put on my shirt, Mary and I were off to the next stop, the medical imaging department, for an X-ray.

Radiography (X-ray)

The X-ray room was simple to find, as it was in the same area where I'd had the bone and CT scans. I checked in at the desk, and within a short time, it was my turn. A nurse asked me to go to the change room, remove all clothing and jewellery, put on a hospital gown and go directly into the medical imaging room. This process required me to pose for a few minutes in front of the X-ray machine, and that was it.

While getting dressed, I was suddenly overwhelmed by emotion. Strangely, I felt depressed at the thought of leaving all the caring people in the hospital and going home, where I'd have nothing to do but wait for the surgery. I'd found the whole hospital experience interesting and soothing.

There was only one more stop, a visit with the anesthesiologist.

THE ANESTHESIOLOGIST

AFTER ASKING FOR DIRECTIONS (yes, I'm learning), we happened upon the anesthesiologist outside of his office. He made us feel welcome. "It's a pleasure to meet you, Gogs," he said with a smile as he vigorously shook my hand. "And you too, Mary," he added while shaking her hand, albeit more gently.

He scored big points there. I had learned in my youth that a firm handshake was a sign of strength, confidence and respect.

"Please come in and have a seat," he invited.

After we sat down, he closed the door, and I handed him the remainder of the paper stack. He reviewed the papers and asked questions about my health very similar to those asked by the pre-admission nurse.

He asked about my previous surgeries. I mentioned the ruptured appendix at age 11 and a few others, including removal of my tonsils, wisdom teeth, gallbladder, several moles and a few lymph nodes from my neck. He made notes and continued to ask questions that I answered to the best of my knowledge.

One of those questions was if I'd ever had any reactions to anesthetics from any surgeries. I said, "No, not really," and went on to describe the day after my wisdom teeth were removed, when my nose wouldn't stop bleeding. I spent the night in the hospital emergency room with an inflated balloon up my nose to stop the bleeding. The culprit was suspected to be a breathing tube that had nicked a blood vessel deep inside the nose canal.

"The old balloon up the nose trick," he replied, smiling. He said a breathing tube wouldn't be needed for my surgery.

He offered a choice between a general or spinal anesthesia. He said that a spinal required fewer drugs and I'd waken with an alert mind, unlike a general which used more drugs and would make me groggy.

He made it clear that the spinal option carried a small risk — about one in 100,000 — of permanent nerve damage around the injection point where he'd guide the needle into my spinal canal. At first, this freaked me out, but I remained calm as he continued to outline the risks and benefits of the two types of anesthesia.

I appreciated the anesthesiologist's honesty, and he earned both Mary's and my trust as he answered our questions. After talking with Mary, I chose the spinal. We favoured using fewer drugs and waking up alert, and our confidence in the doctor overshadowed any worry about potential risks.

He asked if I was allergic to any medications. "Just codeine," I replied and explained how just one drop would put me in the emergency room with an extremely sharp chest pain, as if a spear had just pierced my heart. The unbearable and constant pain would remain until I was given a concoction named a 'pink lady' — not the alcoholic drink but a powerful antacid. One tablespoon is all it would take to alleviate the pain within half a minute.

I first discovered this allergy as a kid, after taking cough medicine with codeine in it. The emergency room doctor who examined me recognized the reaction, brought me the pink drink and alerted me to stay away from codeine. Years later, it happened again by accident, and I've been extra careful to keep clear of it ever since.

The anesthesiologist took notes and assured me nothing would contain codeine.

He began to discuss the upcoming prostate cancer surgery. Although already familiar with the process based on my research and discussions with the urologist, I asked him to spare no details. His face lit up with a big smile, and he leaned towards me from his chair and laid out the entire surgical process.

During his explanation, it became clear that he too shared a deep passion for his work, similar to my urologist, and it struck a chord. I had a good feeling about my health-care team.

The anesthesiologist took time to put in plain words everything and encouraged questions, which further increased our confidence in him. His explanation of the open radical retropubic prostatectomy procedure confirmed my understanding, and it was helpful to review.

Basically, my prostate would be removed through an incision in the lower abdomen the old-fashioned way — with human hands. The surgeon cuts a three-inch incision from the pubic area halfway to the navel, separates the abdominal muscles, cuts the prostate from the bladder and urethra, removes the prostate and then attaches the bladder directly to the urethra.

Of everything he talked about, the two most intriguing aspects to me were pain and blood loss.

In terms of rating pain on a scale of 1 to 10, the anesthesiologist assessed the radical retropubic prostatectomy surgery as a five. That rating didn't sound too bad, although it was hard to relate to, since it was so conceptual. However, I was glad it wasn't higher up on the scale.

Regarding blood loss, he said, "Radical retropubic prostatectomy is a very bloody operation." During the procedure, apparently, it's normal to lose a pint or two of blood.

"You see, Gogs, the prostate is located deep inside the pelvis," he said, and added that it's surrounded by other organs and structures that are vulnerable to injury, such as the rectum, the bladder, the sphincter responsible for urinary control, large blood vessels and the nerves that control erections. However, he assured me there'd be spare blood available if needed and praised the professionalism of my surgical team.

After he answered all our questions, I was ready to proceed with confidence. Mary confirmed her approval to move forward. We thanked him and shook his hand.

Although I didn't say it out loud, the words "Bring it on" came to mind. For some reason, that expression gave me strength.

After five hours in the hospital and nothing more on the to-do list, we felt relieved and accomplished. To celebrate this significant milestone, we treated ourselves to fine dining at a local upscale restaurant and enjoyed an evening on the town. It was a wonderful finale to our pre-surgical time in the hospital.

PREPARING YOUR WILL

EVERYBODY SHOULD WRITE a will of estate while they can to avoid creating problems for others. Even though there wasn't a high risk of death from the surgery or the prostate cancer, I'd learned in Boy Scouts always to "be prepared." Knowing my final wishes were legally documented gave me major peace of mind.

Preparing a will isn't necessarily a sign of affluence (especially for me). It simply helps your survivors deal with your death. That was the main reason for updating my will — to spare my family any legal complications resulting from a lack of planning on my part. Your planning should include what to do with your assets and liabilities and what to do in the event you are no longer medically capable of making rational decisions.

There is a lot of information available on preparing a will, from books, the internet, legal institutions and notary publics. Please take the time to ensure your final wishes are legally documented.

CHAPTER FIVE

SURGERY

Sometimes one must cut off a finger to save a hand.

— Master Po speaking to Caine
   Dialogue from the TV series Kung Fu, "Pilot"
   episode, 1972

The Waiting Game

WAITING THE NEXT FOUR WEEKS for surgery wasn't as stressful as the previous month's wait for the results of the second prostate biopsy. It was a void. No more tests, no more results, no more research and no more extensive talks with family, friends and other prostate cancer survivors. Mary and I were pleased with the surgeon and anesthesiologist and the decision to proceed with surgery. All risks and potential side effects were accepted, mental and physical preparation was done, and it was back to business as usual.

For anyone considering treatment — regardless of whether it's surgery, radiation or other options — please ensure you trust and have confidence in your health-care team and they have extensive successful experience in their field. In my opinion, the number of procedures performed by your team is only part of the equation. Ideally, they should have a proven track record, with many patients experiencing good recovery. We've all heard the cliché "practice makes perfect." However, my martial arts training background has taught me that *only perfect practice makes perfect*. In other words, quality is far more important than quantity.

As the days and weeks passed, I kept busy working as a computer programmer, doing chores around the house, writing notes in the journal and spending quality time with family and dogs. It was a pleasant surprise to accomplish many items on the to-do list while thinking less about the upcoming surgery. Keeping busy was healthy and rewarding.

Inspirational Surprise

A FEW DAYS BEFORE THE SURGERY, Mary and I were out on a daily neighbourhood walk with the dogs. We've always taken the same route and have become friends with many neighbours. Our dogs have met every other dog or cat and know where they all live.

During this walk, we saw our neighbour Roy driving our way. He honked, pulled over and shouted, "How the heck are you guys?" adding with a big chuckle, "I was just thinking about you."

"Roy!" I said enthusiastically. We exchanged greetings and caught up on the latest news.

When I told Roy I was scheduled to have prostate cancer surgery in a few days, he pointed at me and retorted, "You're kidding! My prostate was removed six months ago!"

This coincidence had all three of us totally surprised. We listened intently as Roy outlined his story from diagnosis to post-surgery. I followed up with several questions and related my story.

Roy really lit up when he found out we had the same surgeon. He grabbed my hand for emphasis as he said the surgeon was fantastic and I'd be in great hands. Hearing him speak so positively about the surgeon — and seeing how good Roy looked and how much energy he had — really boosted my confidence.

Roy is a bit older than me and in awe-inspiring shape. He dances several times a week and is always upbeat, positive and on the go. It was hard to fathom that he looked and felt so energetic despite having had his prostate removed only six months before. On top of that, his recovery from side effects was going exceptionally well.

None of the prostate cancer survivors I'd interviewed had had such a recent experience, and only some of them had opted for surgery over other treatments. Therefore, it was captivating to hear about his experience.

As we waved goodbye, I said, "You probably won't see us out here next week."

To our surprise, he snapped, "I don't see why the heck not!"

The talk really energized us, and we continued our walk with an extra pep in our step.

"Bring on the surgery!" I announced to the world.

OPERATING ROOM

IT WAS SURGERY DAY. Could the cancer really have been diagnosed only less than two months ago? Getting to this point had been stressful and sometimes overwhelming. I wouldn't have fared as well without Mary's constant support — it truly was a blessing to have her by my side. We were in good spirits, but we knew this was only the beginning.

We had followed the pre-operation instructions closely for two weeks. No vitamins, herbs, glucosamine, fish oils, ginseng, garlic, aspirin or meat of any kind were consumed. With daily exercise, and holding off on the junk food, I returned to my ideal weight of 185 pounds, and I was mentally and physically prepared for the surgery.

The day started early. At 5:00 a.m., I removed my wedding ring, showered using a chlorhexidine sponge,[12] put on a hospital wristband, grabbed the overnight pack and drove to the hospital with Mary and the kids for a 6:15 a.m. check-in. The sun was rising, and it was as if we were heading out on vacation. However, this trip seemed surreal. We didn't see anyone or anything — it was dead quiet everywhere. As we neared the hospital, it was tempting to drive past and make a run for it, but the car turned into the hospital parking lot despite my thoughts of escape.

We purchased a three-day parking pass, walked in through the main entrance to the administration desk and proceeded to check in. Things seemed to be in slow motion, and the administration clerk's voice sounded distorted.

The clerk instructed us to follow the trail of red dots on the floor to the surgical waiting room. As we waited there, other patients arrived with family and friends, who all looked solemn or worried. Mary and I held hands and watched the clock on the wall while our kids browsed through magazines. Whenever the sound of approaching footsteps was heard, everyone would look up to see if it was their turn.

After 20 minutes a nurse called my name and escorted us to another room. She asked me to change into a hospital gown and lie on the bed. She checked my blood pressure and said it shouldn't be too much

---

12   The antibacterial compound in the chlorhexidine sponge helps reduce germs on your skin and lowers the risk of infection at the surgical site. Please be sure to follow the instructions provided by your health-care team.

longer until surgery. I suddenly grasped that this was reality. Surgery would happen — soon.

After the nurse left the room, Mary reassured us that everything was going to be okay. We remained calm and tried to enjoy the moment and take things slowly. According to the clock on the wall, we had 15 more minutes. Mary and I held hands and talked about celebrating after the operation.

The nurse returned rather quickly with a porter. The surgery was ahead of schedule. She asked me to say goodbye to the family. It was a sudden and abrupt end to our wait. As the porter wheeled me away, Mary shed a few tears, and I looked away to avoid doing the same.

I waved to Mary and the kids until they disappeared from sight. The porter wheeled me down a long hallway, through doorways and a few turns, parking me in a waiting area next to the operating room. I looked around but saw no other patients. It struck me that the operation would be soon.

The clock on the wall seemed unusually loud as it ticked away. Several hospital staff walked about — some smiled while others rushed. The surgeon and anesthesiologist appeared and greeted me with friendly faces. I was pleased to see them, and the surgeon said they'd be ready for me soon. As they went into the operating room, a nurse approached and asked me to get up and to follow them in. (The lack of full service was somewhat disappointing.) I got off the bed and followed her into the room. My hands trembled, my heart pounded, my legs were heavy — the walk was dreadful. The phrase 'dead man walking' recurred to me, but this time the feeling was more intense.

The operating room was very bright and much cooler than the hallway, which didn't help my shaking. The surgeon greeted me and introduced his surgical team: five people all wearing scrubs, hats and masks. That sight was unsettling enough, but when I saw a tray full of shiny surgical knives and a lineup of other scary-looking tools, my knees buckled a bit, and it felt as if the blood was draining from my body.

The nurse asked me to sit on the edge of a narrow operating table in the centre of the room and held me as the anesthesiologist injected the sedative and did the spinal. I felt a small prick in my lower back and quickly became drowsy. The nurse held me tighter as my body became limp and she laid me on the table. She put a blood-pressure cuff on my right arm, and the anesthesiologist hooked up an intravenous on my left arm. I looked up at him with blurred vision as he said, "Don't worry, Gogs, this will all be over before you know it."

This time I didn't have the strength to say, "Bring it on!"

SAYING GOODBYE TO PROSTATE

THE LAST THING I SAW was a bright set of overhead lights moving in and forcing me to close my eyes. Then it was lights out.

While I was completely sedated, my body parts had another imaginary serious conversation.

Prostate: This is it, fellas. It truly was an honour and a privilege to be your friend all these years. And please, no sad faces.

Penis: I'm going to miss you terribly. I can't imagine life without you.

Rectum: You were the best, Prostate. You never caused any trouble. It's not fair.

Prostate: Listen, fellas, it's time to think about yourselves. I've had a good life, helped father three wonderful children. My time's up, that's all.

Penis: We've always been together and made a great team. This is so sad.

Rectum: You've been a true friend, Prostate.

Prostate: Listen carefully, fellas, it's important for you to stay strong without me. You're going to need all the strength you can muster to recover from surgery, and it won't be easy going. Promise me you'll stay strong and not be sad when I'm gone. Be grateful for our time together and remember the good times. Promise me!

Rectum: I promise.

Penis: I promise, too.

Prostate: That's the spirit, fellas. I'm counting on you to live your life to the fullest. Just because my life ends doesn't mean yours does, too.

Penis: Life won't be the same without you.

Rectum: We'll miss you.

Prostate: Fellas, focus on yourselves and your recovery.

Rectum, you'll be sore for many weeks, perhaps months. Don't strain with that first bowel movement. It'll be like a waterslide without water — lots of frustration, pain and very little movement. Avoid food that's hard to digest or produces gas. And take a mild laxative every day until you regain your strength. Rectum, say you'll do this for me.

Rectum: I will, Prostate. You can count on it.

Prostate: Penis, you'll get the worst of it. The surgery will knock out your wind for months, possibly longer. You'll suffer leakage and have problems standing up. I know you've been doing Kegel[13] exercises and those will help tremendously with your recovery. Penis, tell me you'll continue with the program.

Penis: I will, Prostate, and I'll never forget you.

Rectum: You're the best, Prostate.

Prostate: Please remember my last words and never give up. You fellas have many more years to enjoy. Make me proud!

> Spock: [Gasping] I have been . . . and always shall be
> . . . your friend. [he places a Vulcan salute on the glass]
> [Gasping] Live long . . . and prosper.
> [Spock dies]
> Kirk: No!
>
> — Dialogue from the movie *Star Trek II: The Wrath of Khan*, 1982

---

13   Kegel exercises strengthen the muscles of the pelvic floor to help regain continence and improve erectile function by squeezing more blood into the penis.

Chapter Six

Post-Surgery

Strength does not come from physical capacity.
It comes from an indomitable will.

— Mahatma Gandhi

Recovery Room

My eyes opened after the best sleep of my life! I woke up completely alert and well rested. I felt amazing and had no pain or discomfort. The anesthesiologist had been right about the spinal anesthesia. Looking around, I observed I'd been moved to the recovery room, but I had no memories of anything.

In a quick body check, I could feel nothing in my mid-section. My knees were bent upwards, held by a tight wrapping around each leg. A nearby nurse asked how I was feeling. I replied, "Great!" and asked about the wrapping. She explained they were compression sleeves to help prevent blood clots. An electric motor pumped air into the sleeves and massaged my legs to improve circulation and keep the blood flowing back to the heart.

She described how to do leg exercises and watched me to ensure they were done correctly. Strangely, my legs moved freely even though I had no feeling in my mid-section. She asked me to breathe deeply and cough to bring up fluid from my lungs to help prevent infection.

As I proceeded with the leg exercises, deep breathing and coughing, the surgeon approached, beaming. He wanted to know how I felt and said the operation had been exceptionally smooth, without complications. He added that my prostate was one of the largest he'd seen. "Impressive," he said.

I laughed out loud, as it's not exactly a body part used to impress others. However, it was a relief to hear there had been no complications and to see the look on his face that showed he was satisfied with the results.

He provided some detail about the surgery, saying I had been on the table for three hours, and the cancer was fairly plentiful, but he was confident it was all removed. He would have a better idea in a week or two after seeing the pathology report.

We shook hands, and I thanked him for a job well done.

Hospital Room

A NURSE WHEELED ME to my hospital room, where my family greeted me with open arms. Mary said the surgeon had said that I was doing fine in the recovery room and a nurse had provided my room number. Being together was a priceless and emotional moment of family support. I'm sure it accelerated my healing process, too.

After about an hour, Mary sensed my exhaustion and left with the kids, planning to return later.

Walkabout

KNOWING EVERYTHING WAS GOOD, I was truly at peace and closed my eyes to catch a few winks.

Then I heard approaching footsteps and looked up to see two nurses standing above me. "Time to get up and walk!" they said.

This was a critical step in recovery for many reasons, including kick-starting the digestive system, clearing out intestinal gas and helping to prevent blood clots developing in the legs and pneumonia in the lungs.

The nurses liberated me from the leg compression sleeves and helped me sit up and rest for a few minutes. With an arm around a nurse on each side, I took a lungful of air and lifted up to stand on my own two feet.

It felt strange when my feet touched the floor for the first time after surgery. My legs responded awkwardly and shook. After a few steps, I was dizzy and asked for help. The nurses held me while I tried to regain my balance. Then they smiled and encouraged me to continue walking.

I walked without support, although slowly and carefully, to the door and continued to the hallway, where a few other patients were walking around or sitting on chairs. I smiled and waved but suddenly felt weak and light-headed. The nurses helped me back to the bed, smiling and encouraging me all the way.

Before the nurses would allow me to sleep, they prepared and injected a needle into my stomach to help prevent blood clots. They said I could expect this injection twice a day, then off they went.

I was feeling good about my walk. It was time for sleep. I stretched my arms and legs, sighed with relief and closed my eyes.

Again, the sound of footsteps neared, and I looked up to see another nurse. She asked if it was a good time to take some blood, to which I laughed and said, "No problem."

I was beginning to realize it might be impossible to get uninterrupted sleep before returning home. While in the hospital after major surgery, there were a lot of protocols and precautions necessary to encourage a full recovery.

Student Nurses

After the blood work, I closed my eyes again, and, just as I was drifting off, a very polite voice interrupted me. A young student nurse introduced herself and her instructor and said she wanted to show me how to clean my urinary catheter and penis.

"Catheter?" I thought. "Oh, that's right, I forgot." During surgery, a flexible plastic tube was inserted into my penis, down my urethra and into my bladder, where it was held in place by a small inflated balloon. The tube allowed urine to drain continuously into a drainage bag that needed to be emptied on a regular basis.

It was vital to learn the proper care and cleaning of the catheter to avoid possible infection, so I welcomed this new visitor. She closed the curtains as I opened my gown, exposing the catheter and penis. It's amazing how your inhibitions disappear while you're under heavy medication in a hospital gown.

At first sight, it was shocking to see a rubber tube coming out of my penis. However, it was just a minor inconvenience on the road to becoming cancer-free, and it would be in place for seven to ten days.

The surgeon had explained at one of the office visits that the urethra travels through the prostate, which is connected to the bladder. Therefore, to remove the prostate, the urethra is cut, and then the prostate is cut and separated from the bladder. Removing it leaves a gap between the bladder and urethra where the prostate used to reside. To fill the gap, the bladder is pulled down and reconnected to the urethra with stitches. The reason for the catheter is to keep this connection dry while the bladder and urethra heal, ensuring it's watertight.

Please note that this is not an easy procedure and you will want to ensure your surgeon has lots of experience and skill. Deciding where to cut the urethra is critical. If the surgeon cuts the urethra too close to the prostate, cancer cells could be left behind. If the urethra is cut too far away, it could damage the sphincter and cause permanent incontinence.

To help with the decision, the surgeons feel for subtle differences in tissue with their gloved fingers. This helps them know exactly where to cut and whether structures next to the prostate are suspicious for cancer. Other techniques are used for laparoscopic and robotic procedures.

As it turned out, there were actually two urinary drainage bags: a larger one for sleeping and a smaller one that would strap to my leg to accommodate better mobility.

The student nurse began to demonstrate the proper cleaning technique as her instructor supervised. As she did this, another young lady poked her head through the curtain. She introduced herself as another student nurse and asked if it was okay to come in and watch. The circumstances had me completely uninhibited, so I gestured for her to come in and said, "No problem."

The student nurses and their instructor were very professional. They impressed me with their knowledge and easy-to-understand instructions for cleaning and changing the two drainage bags.

Just as they were finishing up, a food service worker brought in a dinner tray. The student nurses and their instructor thanked me for the experience and said they'd give me privacy to eat. That seemed humorous, especially after that very personal demonstration.

I thanked them, said goodbye, looked at the tray and saw a liquid dinner.

> I'm at the age where food has taken the place of sex in my life. In fact, I've just had a mirror put over my kitchen table.
>
> — Rodney Dangerfield

While enjoying my private repast, I felt fortunate to be surrounded by medical professionals who were very caring, warm and exceptional people.

Night Plight

SHORTLY AFTER I ATE — in reality, drank — dinner, Mary and the kids returned for an evening visit, bringing cards and small gifts. Mary hugged and kissed me. They were pleased to see I was looking and feeling good, which for a minute made me want to return home. But my stay was booked for at least two nights, possibly more, depending on my progress.

After a few hours of visiting, it was time to get some much-needed sleep. We said our goodbyes, and it seemed a perfect ending to a perfect day.

The day wasn't quite over, however. The surgeon popped in for a visit around 10:30 p.m. I was astonished he was still in the hospital after such an early start, as it was now about 15 hours later. He was on his way home and wanted to check on me. I replied that I felt great and was pleased with the care and attention from the nurses. He was glad to hear it, and after talking for a few minutes, I thanked him again for a job well done, and we said our goodbyes.

In the night, I became restless and bothered from body heat resulting from the leg compression sleeves, and my lower back was sore from lying on it too long. It was awkward and painful to roll over as I tried to get some relief and find a comfortable position to sleep.

Suddenly, there was a sharp pain in the tip of my penis. I rang for the night nurse, who first opened the window to address the heat and then provided some much-needed pain medication. She suggested the penis pain was due to surgery and inserting the catheter, and should get better over time. In the meantime, she continued to check up on me every hour, giving me more pills every four hours throughout the entire night.

Her help and dedication were much appreciated. However, the pain always returned before the next dose of medication.

On the 1 to 10 pain scale, the soreness in my back scored a 6, the sharp pain in the tip of my penis was an 8, and the pain from the incision was a mere one.

During the night, the nurse helped to reposition me a few times using pillows. This would provide temporary relief and bring the pain under control, but I couldn't fall asleep. Whatever the reason, I simply didn't sleep a wink all night.

Unexpected Closure

The anesthesiologist visited me in the early morning of May 2 and asked about my pain. He had heard about the sleepless night and was concerned. I was happy to say that the pain from my incision was extremely low. However, my back was sore, and the real predicament was the pain in the tip of my penis.

He was relieved about the mild incision pain and thought that the penis pain was most likely due to the catheter rubbing on the tip. He said he'd talk to the nurse about it. I thanked him for the visit and anticipated further pain relief.

A short while later, the two student nurses and their instructor returned. It was a pleasure to see them, as I felt very well looked after and safe under their care.

Today's lessons were the proper care and cleaning of the incision and how to empty the surgical drain.

"Oh, the surgical drain," I thought. Another item I'd forgotten.

The anesthesiologist had talked about this during the pre-admission appointment. There are two incisions made during surgery. One is the main incision in the lower abdomen through which the prostate is removed. The other is a much smaller incision close to the main incision, where the surgical drain tube is inserted. Free-floating on the inside, the tube is held in place by a stitch in the lower abdomen and secured with removable tape.

The part of the tube on the outside is connected to a small removable container. Before attaching the container, you squeeze the air out of it. Once connected, it slowly fills with air and creates a vacuum. The purpose is to drain stray blood and other fluids left over from surgery. Eventually, the container refills and needs to be disconnected, emptied, re-squeezed and reconnected. The surgical drain is usually removed a few days after surgery. When it's time to remove it, you simply cut the stitch, pull the tube out and cover the small incision with a bandage.

Before the cleaning, I confided in the student nurses, telling them about the unbearable pain in the tip of my penis. The instructor left the room and quickly returned with a tube of numbing jelly. A few minutes after it was applied, the pain subsided and I felt much better and ready for the demonstration.

During the cleaning, the nurses expressed interest in hearing my story. I told them how being diagnosed with prostate cancer had impacted my life, starting with how it had not been easy to accept. I talked about how researching it and journaling my thoughts and feelings throughout the process had helped me to accept the situation and build the confidence to move forward and opt for surgery.

The nurses listened intently and were very supportive. I mentioned my sister's passing in 2010 from ovarian cancer at the age of fifty-six. "Joanne was my best friend," I said.

Sharing this reminded me how hard it was for her and the family during the last year of chemotherapy, especially her final days in hospice. I was with her during her final moments as her arms and legs twitched involuntarily. At that point, I finally confessed to being the one who had hidden — and later eaten — her wedding cake[14] in 1976. The look on her face was priceless as she first grinned and then laughed. I held her hand, kissed her forehead and said, "I love you."

These thoughts brought back a flood of memories, and suddenly I became overwhelmed with emotion and cried uncontrollably.

---

14 Joanne had two wedding cakes, both vanilla with royal white icing covered with red roses. The main cake was beautifully displayed on a classic three-tier structure and used for the traditional cake-cutting ceremony and to serve guests. The second, dome-shaped cake was to allow for extra servings. This is the cake I hid and later ate in just under a week's time. My conscience is grateful that I finally confessed.

During the breakdown, I thought about Joanne's and my childhood and our other sister, Brenda, who passed away from a rare heart disorder at the age of 20 months — eight months before I was born. I had always wondered what it would have been like to have another sister in my life, and now, once again, I grieved her loss.

The nurses were extremely compassionate. They held my hands, rubbed my shoulders and cheered me up with very kind words. I regained control and confessed that it's hard to always play the tough guy, and telling them about it made me feel healthier. They urged me to get some rest, as I hadn't slept since waking up in the recovery room about 26 hours earlier. I was overtired and emotionally drained.

The nurses promised to return later, and I waved goodbye. Then I closed my eyes and contemplated both their kindness and the emotional breakdown I had just experienced.

After some thought, I realized it was caused by feelings of mourning over the loss of my sister that I had held inside for the past seven years. The breakdown had brought an incredible emotional release that made me feel elated, stronger, completely pain-free and entirely at peace.

> Dr. Leonard H. "Bones" McCoy: The release of emotions, Mr. Spock, is what keeps us healthy — emotionally healthy, that is.
>
> — Dialogue from the TV series *Star Trek*, "Plato's Step children" episode, 1968

Unstoppable Force

Before I had time to fall asleep, a nurse arrived and asked if I had been passing gas. It was funny to realize the hospital might be the only place that applauds flatulence. Perhaps there should be a bell hanging from the ceiling with a rope you can pull when passing gas. I imagined ringing the bell and seeing people running from every direction to congratulate and cheer.

Jokes aside, passing gas is a healthy sign indicating the bowels are returning to normal after surgery. Unfortunately, I hadn't passed gas or had a bowel movement since surgery. Both are important signs indicating the digestive system is awake and functioning. Without these signs, the surgeon is likely to restrict you to a liquid diet. This was apparent when my lunch was served, and again, it was all liquid. It was disappointing, as I was hungry and really wanted to sink my teeth into something, but I understood the reasoning for the restriction.

After the liquids, I felt much stronger and was itching for another walkabout. I rang for the nurse, who came and removed the leg compression sleeves and helped me stand. From there, I was off, out the door, down the hallway and moving exceptionally well.

During the second lap around the hallway, I had a strong urge to pass gas. It suddenly turned into a powerful, unstoppable force that usually I would try to conceal. However, being in the hospital, where it's considered a good thing, I decided to just let 'er rip.

"Uh-oh!" I said. "I hope that was just air." It was a relief, whatever it was, but it had hurt my rectum, caused a sharp pain in my lower back and flexed my abdominals, which pulled on the incision, causing more pain.

I stood motionless for a few seconds, trying to detect anything new out back while looking around to see if anybody had noticed. On my third breath, my senses detected bad air, which was no longer breathable. I rushed back to my room, where I hid in the washroom and tried to have a bowel movement. Passing solids rather than gas could be my real meal ticket. However, even after sitting for a while, nothing happened.

As I exited the washroom, a nurse entered and said it was time for the stomach needle. She asked if I had had a bowel movement or passed any gas.

I paused, and for the good of my health, I disclosed ownership of the major gas leak in the hallway.

"That was you?" she responded as my face turned beet-red and hot.

She helped me into bed, reconnected the compression sleeves and injected the blood-clot prevention medication.

As I gave a thumbs-up and waved goodbye, another nurse entered. It was time for more blood work. I don't think I ever did get to sleep. But I wasn't about to complain. The level of care was exceptional, and I felt fortunate to be under the supervision of such fantastic health-care professionals.

SURPRISE VISIT

LATER IN THE AFTERNOON, a doctor entered and introduced himself as the assistant surgeon. The pre-admission nurse had said he often worked on my surgeon's team, and I figured that any friend of my surgeon was undoubtedly a friend of mine. We had met during the introductions in the operating room, but he'd been wearing a mask and my mind had been somewhat preoccupied.

He said the team was extremely pleased with the outcome of the surgery and commented that my prostate was the largest he'd ever seen. "Hmmm," I thought, "this would make a good rocking-chair story."

Old Grandpa Gogs: In my day, I had one of the biggest prostates ever seen by man. It took two surgeons to carry it to the pathology lab. Today, it sits under glass in the medical hall of fame.

The assistant surgeon concluded with the encouraging news that I could be released in the morning. We shook hands, and I thanked him for his visit.

FAMILY VISIT

WITHOUT QUALITY SLEEP in more than 30 hours, I felt surprisingly awake and alert, likely due to the news that my vital signs and blood work were normal. Knowing

I could be returning home in the morning had me revved up, and I was also looking forward to another planned visit from Mary and the kids.

A nurse entered and said it was time for another stomach needle. Being pumped, I asked for another walkabout. After the shot, she removed the sleeves, helped me stand, and off I went into the hallway, where I walked around and talked with other patients. Before long, Mary and the kids arrived. After I shared the good news of my potential release in the morning, we returned to the room to continue our discussions on post-surgery celebrations.

They visited until dinner arrived. Liquid again. It consisted of a cup of beef broth, a bowl of red gelatin, a cup of coffee and a glass of apple juice. Certainly not enough to fill me up, although I was grateful for the meal and understood that eating anything more could cause complications if my digestive system wasn't yet fully activated.

Hospital Release

The date was May 3, 2017. During the previous night, my sleep had been interrupted by the return of the sharp pain in the tip of my penis. This time the tube of numbing jelly was close at hand and I applied it myself. Not all men have trouble with the catheter, but for me, it was brutally painful and inconvenient, as it reminded me of its presence every time my body moved.

After another liquid breakfast, a nurse let me know that the surgeons had approved my release, and that she had already informed my family. She freed me from the leg compression sleeves. Then she cut the stitch that anchored the surgical drain tube and pulled it out. It was a lot longer than I'd expected, and its removal stung for a few seconds. On the pain scale, it was only a three out of ten. The nurse explained that the stitches in my incision were dissolvable and the small strips of tape covering them would fall off on their own. A large bandage covered the incision, stitches and tape. It would need to be changed, and the area cleaned, every day.

Within a short time, Mary and the kids arrived. I put on my robe, gathered my belongings and sat in the wheelchair. As Mary wheeled me out, the nurses, including the student nurses and their instructor, all said goodbye and wished me well.

Although it felt liberating to be returning home, it was sad to leave the care of such wonderful people and realize I might not see them again.

CHAPTER SEVEN

HOME RECOVERY

If you even dream of beating me you'd better wake
up and apologize.

— Muhammad Ali

HOME SWEET HOME

ON THE DRIVE HOME, I looked out the window,
appreciating everything in sight. It no longer bothered
me to be stuck behind slow drivers or cut off by
someone in a hurry. I genuinely enjoyed every moment
as it unfolded. I had gained a new respect for life. It's
true that the simple things in life are pure gold and not
to be taken for granted.

As we pulled into the driveway, the surgery seemed like a dream. Memories of being on the operating table seemed distant, almost forgotten. Our house looked very inviting, and it was uplifting to know we would be inside soon.

As we opened the front door, our two dogs immediately rushed to greet us, and I had to guard my incision and catheter. The dogs could easily knock me over, or worse, pull on the catheter. They sniffed up and down continuously with their eyes wide open. They were probably wondering if I'd brought them a treat.

I sat on the couch, leaned back and took a deep breath, thinking, "It's hard to believe the surgery's already over and I'm home." I was in absolutely no pain or discomfort of any kind. Even the tip of my you-know-what was pain-free. I just sat there in high spirits while the dogs took their usual spot on the floor.

Mary prepared a light lunch, which was a step up from the liquid diet. She diligently ensured that I drank 10 to 12 cups of water throughout the day. She also made sure I walked. At first it was just a few laps around the hallway, with the goal to return to our regular routine of walking the dogs.

Overall, it was a great day and fantastic to be home.

After a full day of spending time with the dogs, walking the hallway, drinking water and eating real food, it was time to call it a night. It was wonderful to stretch out in bed, and I was looking forward to finally getting some much-needed, long-overdue sleep.

FAINTING EPISODE

THE NEXT MORNING, I woke up rested after managing to get some sleep. However, I was still unable to roll to either side, and my lower back ached. I sat up on the edge of the bed and Mary provided major relief as she massaged my back. Within a few minutes, the soreness improved.

Ready to greet the day, I noticed the drainage bag needed to be emptied. When I lifted it, I realized it was quite heavy when close to full and I had to be careful. I had taken this for granted in the hospital, as the nurses always emptied it. This morning, it seemed like a hassle. However, the truth was that I missed the attention of all the nurses.

After emptying it, then showering and getting dressed, it was time for a few laps around the hallway.

I started strong and was feeling positive. However, I must have been pushing too hard, because all of a sudden, my energy was zapped dry. I barely had enough strength to alert my son, Alex: "I'm going to fall."

Luckily for me, Alex is a health-care worker and he stepped up to the plate. He managed to prevent the fall and get me safely back into bed. Then he removed my bathrobe and instructed Mary to rub a cold facecloth on my forehead while he took my blood pressure, which was 116 over 70. After a few minutes, it returned to 120 over 80.

Mary called the urologist and left a message with his receptionist. Within 20 minutes he called back, asked several questions, reminded me to take it easy and said to call 911 if it happened again.

However, he repeated an earlier warning not to allow anyone — not even another urologist, doctor or nurse — to remove the catheter, even in an emergency. He made it clear that the catheter was carefully positioned with regard to my specific radical prostatectomy, and it must not be removed or replaced by anyone who did not perform the surgery.

I took comfort in his calm nature and guidance. Deep down inside, I just wanted to return to normal as quickly as possible. But I had to admit that even though my mind was ready, my body still needed more time.

I reminded myself of the hospital release rules. No driving for two weeks, no vigorous activity or lifting more than five pounds for six weeks, no climbing stairs, no sitting longer than 45 minutes at a time, no sexual activity for six weeks and no pools or bathtubs with the catheter. In the meantime, showers only.

From that point forward, I decided I was going to be the model prostate cancer survivor and make my urologist proud. I'd adjust my thinking and change my mindset. Rather than focusing on the end goal of full recovery, I made a mental note to aim for smaller, more manageable goals that would serve as stepping stones to the end result.

EMERGENCY ROOM

Shortly after that conversation with the urologist, I had a super-strong urge to have a bowel movement. This would be my first one since the prostatectomy, and I had been instructed not to strain, especially so soon after surgery.

There was nothing to do other than head for the washroom, relax and let nature take its course.

It's actually a bit awkward sitting on a toilet with a catheter. I had to be watchful not to step on or pull the tube and carefully handle the drainage bag, all while holding on to my incision.

I did my best not to strain. However, the urge was overpowering, and as a result, I experienced a bladder spasm. This is when the bladder muscle squeezes suddenly without warning, causing an urgent need to release urine.

In my case, it caused the balloon that holds the catheter in place to shift, allowing urine to run uncontrollably down the urethra and thus escape on the outside of the catheter tube and onto the floor. When the urine flowed over the stitches where the bladder was connected to the urethra, it caused a burning sensation.

Also, my lower back was sore, there was a sharp pain deep inside my rectum, and the pain from the incision reached level 6 out of 10 on the pain scale.

Captain James T. Kirk: Perhaps man wasn't meant for paradise. Maybe he was meant to claw, to scratch all the way.

— Dialogue from the TV series *Star Trek*, "This Side of Paradise" episode, 1967

That's when it happened: my first bowel movement since surgery. It completely drained all energy. I immediately felt sick and weak, with a strong urge to pass out. I called Mary, who called 911. While we waited, she rubbed my back and said everything was going to be okay.

An ambulance arrived within 15 minutes. Mary flagged it down and escorted in two very tall, muscular men. They calmly and swiftly began to assess my health and vital signs. As they worked, they smiled and asked several questions. With my blood pressure even lower than before — 110 over 60 — they decided to take me to emergency.

The whole experience was a bit of a blur. I don't remember getting into the ambulance, but I recall it was immaculate and modern, with a bunch of fancy gizmos and gadgets. I faded in and out, and it seemed like by the time I blinked, we had already arrived at the hospital.

The ambulance workers helped me outside, where a nurse was waiting with a wheelchair. Once we were inside, she hooked me up to a portable heart rate monitor and proceeded to ask first me and then the ambulance workers several questions.

All of a sudden, the alarm on the monitor rang as my blood pressure dropped to 100 over 40. Almost immediately, they rushed me into an emergency room, and five or six medical professionals surrounded me. One put an intravenous into my left arm, and another took some blood out of my right arm, while another looked me in the eye and continued to say my name: "Gogs, stay awake, Gogs, stay with me, Gogs."

I was lifted onto a hospital bed. I remember attempting to speak, nervous they might remove the catheter. I tried to tell them, but the words were either incomprehensible or too quiet to hear.

Mary and the kids arrived about 15 minutes later. My natural instinct was to play the tough guy and tell them everything was okay. However, I have learned that this behaviour can bottle up unresolved emotions, which may explode later in life. Therefore, I reached for Mary's hand, looked deep into her eyes and said, "I love you."

After being on the intravenous for about an hour, I felt much better and more alert. My blood pressure had returned to 120 over 80. The emergency doctor said my blood work looked good — the fainting episode was most likely due to vasovagal syncope, which is a temporary fall in blood pressure causing a lack of blood to the brain.

Emergency Doctor: "We get a lot of old guys in here that have fainted after having a big bowel movement." He then made a fainting gesture.

I laughed out loud, but paused and thought, "Old guy? I'm only fifty-seven." I sure hope that's not how it will end for me. I can just imagine the eulogy at my funeral: "With his final breath, he left behind a massive and impressive bowel movement."

Catheter Woes

THE DAY AFTER BEING RELEASED from emergency, I called the urologist to give him an update. He reminded me that I should be taking a mild laxative every day and not eating food that was difficult to digest. After all, it had only been five days since the surgery. Not only was I pushing too hard, I had also returned to my usual diet way too soon. Due to my fainting episodes, he made the decision to leave the catheter in place for a few additional days.

Again, his calm nature helped me realize that I needed to focus and take recovery more earnestly in order to be the model prostate cancer survivor.

• • •

During the following ten days, all I could think about was getting rid of the catheter. It was a real drag — cleaning, draining and carrying the drainage bags. Changing from one bag to the other and back again. Having to be mindful while sleeping, sitting, walking, showering and using the washroom. Keeping the drainage bag lower than my bladder to ensure proper urine flow — making sure always to protect my penis and catheter. I had a fear the drainage tube would get caught or tangled around something and get yanked out unexpectedly, causing pain and internal damage that might lead to permanent incontinence. Also, I had to keep applying the numbing jelly regularly to relieve the sharp pain in the tip of my penis.

Again, I had to keep reminding myself that the catheter was just a minor inconvenience and not a big deal in the grand scheme of things. It's easy to get hung up on small matters and lose perspective of the more important picture. After all, it was only a few weeks out of my entire life, and to become cancer-free was well worth the price.

Other than my frustration with the catheter, recovery had been going remarkably well. I was no longer taking any pain medication, and I was back to walking the dogs with Mary.

I was sleeping through the night with the help of the catheter. That was the positive side of the extra plumbing — no need to get up to pee. And as a bonus, my lower back was no longer sore, so I could roll over in bed during the night. Generally speaking, I was doing great.

Here I wish to acknowledge my two daughters, Stacey and Jenn, for always being there to assist with daily tasks. I would not have managed so well without their support during this part of recovery.

Removing the Catheter

It was May 15, the appointment date to remove the catheter. I was so excited that while changing from the larger bag to the smaller leg bag, I forgot to pinch the hose and some urine leaked out onto the floor. I was literally making a mess of things. I must have made this change dozens of times, but today I was having trouble.

After a few more minutes of struggling, I finally got the connections right. However, I became aware that while I was walking, the tube kept pulling on my penis — the leg bag wasn't strapped in the right place. After a quick adjustment, Mary drove us to the urologist's office. I was so excited that you would have thought I'd just won the lottery. I couldn't wait to be free of this apparatus, and not only because it was a major pain. It was a significant milestone in recovery.

We arrived in record time, and it was heartening to see the ladies at the administration desk, as they were always smiling and helpful. I checked in, took a seat and waited. After a short while, the urologist greeted us with a handshake.

Mary and I followed him into the office, where we talked about my progress. I was happy to report everything was going well — but so impatient to get on with it that I hopped up onto the table in mid-conversation.

The urologist laughed and put on a pair of gloves. We continued our discussions while he used a syringe to drain the catheter balloon. Once it was deflated, he simply pulled the tube out and threw everything into a bin. It was quick and painless. Just an odd, fleeting sensation and I instantly felt a whole lot better. Now that I was no longer restricted by the tube, my mobility would improve dramatically.

He said not to get up until he got a diaper. "Okay," I said, still wondering about leakage. I had no idea if all the Kegel exercises I'd done up until the surgery had paid off or not. However, after investigating, I was pleasantly surprised to see everything was dry and seemed quite normal.

When the urologist gave me the diaper, I was totally stunned by the look and feel. It didn't look anything like a diaper from the old days. Even the colour threw me: light gray, very modern. And it looked just like underwear. As I put it on, it was amazingly comfortable and supportive, which was a major relief. I had not been looking forward to wearing such a product.

After pulling my pants up over my modern underwear, I eased myself off the table and immediately had an intense burning sensation in the tip of my penis. I quickly realized the burning was caused by a leak of a few drops of urine. Thank goodness for the modern underwear — nobody would be the wiser.

With that, we both shook his hand and thanked him for everything. On the way out, Mary and I decided to celebrate this key milestone in recovery by visiting a tattoo parlour. We had both talked about this for years, and although it was fun to look, we didn't go through with it that day (and still haven't yet). Instead, we took a romantic walk along the beach before going out for dinner and a movie.

ANXIOUSLY AWAITING

DURING THE FOLLOWING THREE DAYS, we stressed about the results of the pathology report. We hadn't heard anything from the urologist, and while no news is usually considered good news, in this case, we needed to know if surgery had removed all the cancer or not.

Meanwhile, it was an absolute pleasure living without the catheter. Simple activities such as walking, sitting, getting in and out of bed and doing chores around the house had become a breeze. I was able to have a real bath and stretch out in bed with the bonus pleasure of rolling over to hug Mary during the night.

On the negative side, I'd been getting up to use the washroom a couple of times a night. I had been counselled to expect this. During surgery, the bladder takes some physical blows, which can make it swell and become irritable. Also, since the catheter had been continuously emptying my urine for the past few weeks, my bladder had shrunk a bit. It would take time to heal and return to its previous size.

However, I was more apprehensive about my weak urine flow. It was a lot worse than it had been before surgery. I consulted the urologist, who thought there could be a possible blockage. He made an appointment for another cystoscopy on May 19. He also mentioned the pathology report would be ready at that time.

In the meantime, I tried not to lose sleep over it, although that was easier said than done.

CHAPTER EIGHT

SURGERY RESULTS

> Difficult roads often lead to beautiful destinations.
> The best is yet to come.
>
> — Zig Ziglar

PATHOLOGY REPORT

ON MAY 19, we met with the urologist. Although the cystoscopy was necessary to check for urethra blockages, it was the pathology report that Mary and I were most anxious about. We checked in at the cystoscopy clinic at the hospital, and a nurse asked me to change into a gown and take a seat in the waiting area. When it was my turn, a nurse escorted me into the examination room and asked me to lie down on the table.

Within a few seconds, the urologist entered. "Hello, Gogs, how are you?"

Being impatient, I replied, "Doing well, what are the results of the pathology report?"

He laughed and said not to worry, as the results were good. However, he was concerned about my weak urine flow.

"Fair enough," I conceded.

After a quick numbing of my urethra, I watched on the monitor as he proceeded to insert the cystoscope into my penis, down my urethra and toward the bladder. I was surprised at how bright the images were. I could see amazing detail.

At one point, he stopped the cystoscope and pointed to the monitor. "See that, Gogs?" he said with excitement. "Those are the stitches where we attached your bladder to your urethra. Your prostate used to be right there." This evoked mixed emotions in me — I was sad that my prostate was gone, but happy the cancer was removed.

He went on to point out that there was no scar tissue forming to get in the way of urine flow and that everything was healing perfectly. After a few more minutes of examining, he said, "Gogs, you're wide open." He meant that there was no physical evidence to account for a weak urine flow. He said that he'd seen this before in other patients. He trusted the flow would improve and asked me to keep him updated.

It was good to know the flow would improve. After he removed the cystoscope, he said, "Okay, Gogs, let's look at that pathology report."

This was the moment of truth. This report had critical details about the extent of the cancer, if it had spread and whether further treatment was necessary.

The urologist explained that during surgery, tissue samples surrounding the prostate are sent to the pathology lab and tested on the spot to determine if more cutting is required. I found it hard to imagine waiting for results while you've got a patient on the table with an open incision, but I'm glad to know it's an efficient process. I figure it's best to get this work done while you're open on the table.

The pathology report confirmed a Gleason score of $4 + 3 = 7$ that had emerged from the second biopsy.

Please note that the pathology report from the prostate biopsy only examines the removed tissue samples, while the pathology report from the surgery examines the entire prostate. Therefore, it's entirely possible for the whole-prostate pathology report to show a higher Gleason than a biopsy does, because a prostate biopsy can find some cancer without finding a more aggressive tumour. In my case, the two pathology reports matched, meaning the earlier prostate biopsy had found the most aggressive tumour.

On the TNM[15] (tumour-node-metastasis) system, the cancer was at stage T2c-N0-M0, bilateral disease, meaning that it had invaded both lobes and was in the

---

15   The TNM system classifies the stage of cancer. T is the size of the primary tumour and describes any local invasion. N indicates whether it has extended or spread to lymph nodes, while M indicates whether it has metastasized to other body parts. In my case, T2c meant cancer had invaded both lobes of the prostate, N0 indicated cancer hadn't spread to the lymph nodes, and M0 showed cancer hadn't spread to other body parts.

final stage before penetrating and escaping the prostate capsule, known as an extraprostatic extension (EPE), independent of the prostate gland. There is no telling how much more time it would have taken until the breach, but I'm glad I had surgery sooner rather than later, as EPE increases the risk of positive surgical margins where cancer can potentially be left behind, requiring radiation therapy after surgery. Or, in efforts to avoid this risk, the surgeon may need to cut wider around the prostate and may possibly end up sacrificing the erection nerves.

At 178.75 cubic centimetres and 5.5 x 6.5 x 5.0 centimetres in dimension, my prostate was nearly three times normal size. It weighed 117 grams and contained 43 percent cancer — a sizable amount. For perspective, my prostate was about the size of four and a half golf balls,[16] of which almost two golf balls were cancer.

The best part of the pathology report was the expression *negative surgical margins*, meaning no cancer cells were found at the outer edge of the removed tissue. In other words, it was likely that no cancerous tissue had been left behind during surgery, and no further treatment would be required at this time.

Needless to say, Mary and I were overjoyed. We hugged each other and shed a few tears. For a few moments, we were both speechless and unable to move, as if we were frozen. Even though this was the

---

16   The average golf ball is 40.973 cubic centimetres. Prostate size divided by golf-ball size (178.75 / 40.973 = 4.36 golf balls). Results multiplied by 43 percent (4.36 x 0.43 = 1.87 golf balls).

news we'd been hoping for, I didn't realize it would hit us just as hard as that first diagnosis had. However, this time the impact was joyful. We were both extremely relieved and hugged the urologist and thanked him for all his support.

Afterwards, we drove home, got into bed and cuddled the rest of the day and throughout the night.

URINARY INCONTINENCE

THE LOSS OF BLADDER CONTROL is a common side effect of radical prostatectomy surgery. In men, there are three layers, or valves, to hold back urine: the internal sphincter, the prostate and the external sphincter. The only one remaining after surgery is the external sphincter, which can be damaged or bruised during the procedure. It may require several weeks or months to recover and heal, depending on your age and how much control you had before the surgery. In some cases — depending on how far the cancer has invaded, the surgical technique and the skill of your surgeon — the external sphincter may be permanently damaged, and you may never regain total control by natural means.[17]

Even though the urologist and anesthesiologist had described the surgery in detail, and I understood there was a risk of permanent incontinence, I didn't fully comprehend what this means: with a prostatectomy,

---

17   In the event you do not regain urinary control, please tell your health-care team.

even in the best-case scenario, you still lose two out of your three urinary valves. Knowing and understanding this fact would have influenced me to weigh my other options more fairly. That said, please be aware that all treatment options carry risks, and it's critical for you to research and discuss with your health-care team.

The external sphincter can hold in urine by itself, but it has to be strong. To prepare for this, I started doing Kegel exercises the same day I was diagnosed with prostate cancer and continued right up until surgery. I stopped while the catheter was in place but resumed them once it was removed, and still do them to this day.

Kegel exercises strengthen the muscles of the pelvic floor, which includes the external sphincter. These are the muscles you squeeze when trying to stop urinating in mid-stream. To perform one repetition, squeeze the muscles around the anus as if you are trying to hold urine or gas. Try to isolate these muscles and do not engage your buttocks, abdominals or any other muscle. Hold for ten seconds and relax. My routine is 20 repetitions, three times a day. However, don't overdo it, as like any muscle, the external sphincter can become fatigued.

Assuming the external sphincter is not permanently damaged, urinary control should return in three distinct phases. The first phase is remaining dry when lying down. For me, this occurred in the first week, so I no longer needed to wear the modern underwear at night.

The second phase is remaining dry when walking around. The real test is being able to walk to the washroom without leaking along the way. That would mean the external sphincter is intact and is an excellent sign. For me, this occurred in the third week. I stopped wearing the modern underwear altogether and started to wear a pad in the daytime only.

The third and final stage is remaining dry while applying pressure on the external sphincter — doing activities such as standing up from a seated position, sneezing, coughing, laughing, stretching, bending, lifting heavy objects or exercising. For me, this occurred in the sixth week. I no longer needed to wear protection of any kind and haven't leaked a drop since.

I attribute a large part of this success to my surgeon and his team for not damaging my external sphincter, the only valve I have left to control urine. The rest I owe to Kegel exercises and the fact that cancer hadn't yet invaded this area.

By the third month, I no longer had to get up during the night to pee, and the force of my urine flow had improved dramatically. It's not quite the same force as in my teens. However, it was a significant improvement over how it had been before surgery. The best part was when, during a shopping trip at a local mall with Mary, I needed to use the public washroom. All the stalls and urinals were occupied except for one urinal. The urge was strong, so I didn't have much choice. I walked up to the vacant urinal, afraid that my bladder shyness would get the best of me. However,

I was pleasantly surprised and had no trouble going. Standing proudly, not caring about the other men and simply doing my business, felt like a victory. Perhaps I was never bladder-shy in the first place, and my difficulty before surgery was most likely a symptom of having prostate cancer.

ERECTILE DYSFUNCTION

THE INABILITY TO GET an erection firm enough for intercourse is a common side effect of radical prostatectomy surgery. The erection nerves, known as the neurovascular bundles (NVB), are like a bundle of wires in an electrical circuit. The two separate nerve bundles run along the surface of each side of the prostate, contained within a layer of tissue called fascia. These bundles need to be delicately separated from the prostate during surgery, which may cause them to be damaged or bruised. Afterwards, they may require several months or years to recover and heal. In some cases, depending on how far cancer has invaded and how large the prostate is, these nerves may have to be removed to ensure no cancer is left behind, and you may never be able to have an erection by natural means.[18]

---

18 A natural erection relies on many factors, including interest, stimulation, testosterone, nerve impulse between the penis and the brain, blood flow into the penis and a healthy heart and circulatory system.

On reflection, I missed out on the opportunity to participate in the Prostate Cancer Supportive Care Program offered by BC Cancer in Victoria. Regardless of your treatment option, they provide comprehensive support that includes managing the impact of prostate cancer treatments on sexual function, intimacy, and rehabilitation. It's never too late, so please consider taking advantage of a program near you.

The only thing I could do was hope the surgeon was able to successfully separate the erection nerves from my prostate with minimal damage. Actually, when the surgeon came to visit in the recovery room, one of my questions was, "Did you save my erection nerves?"

He wasn't surprised by the question, as it's a common concern and he gets asked all the time. I was happy and relieved to hear that he'd been able to spare the erection nerves. However, he warned that it might take several months or years before I regained a natural erection.

Before the surgery, he had explained that erection and orgasm are two separate and different functions, and losing one doesn't necessarily mean you lose the other. In other words, you don't need an erection to have an orgasm, in the same way you don't need an orgasm to have an erection. (I had actually already learned this fact back in 1972 as a kid going through puberty with a big collection of *Playboy* magazines.)

However, I lost a few things with the surgery. Since my prostate and seminal vesicles have been removed, I'm no longer able to father children and will never again experience ejaculation. (Although semen is still produced in the testicles, it's simply reabsorbed into the body, and the orgasms are dry.) This loss actually increases my sexual drive, as now there's no fear of impregnation. This gives me a sense of freedom to be promiscuous in my dreams, like James Bond, one of my heroes when I was growing up. I used to fantasize about what it would be like to be a top-ranking British intelligence officer armed with a license to kill — and an international playboy making out with beautiful women from around the world.

James Bond: Miss Anders! I didn't recognise you with your clothes on.

— Dialogue from the movie *The Man with the Golden Gun*, 1974

After surgery, my penis showed no signs of life for a good three months. That is, until one night during deep sleep, when a pulsing from down below awakened me. My eyes opened wide in disbelief and I thought maybe it was a dream. That's when it happened: my penis started moving about as if awakening from a long, lifeless slumber. He stretched out and continued to pulse for a few short minutes. Then he curled up and fell asleep again.

Typically, the average healthy male will have three to five erections during sleep. Having nightly erections is an excellent sign the body is working and indicates that erectile dysfunction symptoms are likely psychological.[19] To determine if nightly erections occur, you might attempt the postage-stamp test. (As a kid, I read many comic books, including *The Incredible Hulk*. Seeing his clothes rip during his transformation into the beast was a thrill. The postage-stamp test reminds me of this process.) You'll need a roll of stamps. Wrap several stamps snugly around the base of the penis, much like a cigar wrapper, and moisten[20] one of the stamps to secure. Put on boxers or briefs to protect the stamps, then go to sleep and dream of the transformation.

> Jack McGee: Forgive me, Doctor., but I am calling you a liar!
>
> Dr. David Banner: Mr. McGee! [Takes a deep breath, smiles] Mr. McGee, don't make me angry. [Chuckles] You wouldn't like me when I'm angry.
>
> — Dialogue from the TV series *The Incredible Hulk*, "Pilot" episode, 1977

Well, you get the picture. And again, this is just a fun test, and it's best to ask your health-care team for more sophisticated analysis.

---

19 Psychological reasons for erectile dysfunction may include stress, performance anxiety and depression, to name just a few. It's best to refer to your health-care team.

20 Or if using self-sticking stamps, peel off the back of one. Just ensure the stamps are perforated.

Even though my erections were slowly returning, I decided to talk to our family doctor about Viagra.[21] She was more than happy to give me a prescription, but asked me to think about intimacy. What if I were to try to remove the pressure of getting an erection and let things happen more naturally? I agreed wholeheartedly. I needed to shift my thinking and change my mindset. Rather than focusing on the erection, I needed to slow down and concentrate my efforts more on romance, intimacy and making a connection with love.[22]

However, since I was curious and had a prescription in hand, it was time to visit the pharmacy. While waiting in line and noticing the pharmacist was a young woman, I imagined her announcing it over the loudspeaker: "We have a prescription for Viagra for Gogs Gagnon."

I thought about leaving. Then I thought about everything that I'd already gone through to get to this point and asked myself, "How embarrassing can it

---

21 Viagra helps improve blood flow to the penis. However, an erection may not occur without other factors such as interest and stimulation. Please speak to your health-care team regarding a variety of ways to achieve an erection, including many types of medication, penis pumps and injections. Be sure to ask about potential side effects and the latest developments.

22 Demonstrating your love for each other by making a mental shift from thinking 'me' to 'we.' Simple is best and might include things like being in the moment, listening, showing respect and appreciation for each other and spending quality time together (date nights with no kids, for example). There are lots of books, information on the internet and relationship counselling available that can do wonders for your love life. Please remember, it's not all about sex.

be?" When she called for me, I proudly handed in the prescription, and within 20 minutes, it was filled.

Armed with the blue pills, I was eager to get home.

> Morpheus: This is your last chance. After this, there is no turning back. You take the blue pill — the story ends, you wake up in your bed and believe whatever you want to believe. You take the red pill — you stay in Wonderland and I show you how deep the rabbit hole goes.

— Dialogue from the movie *The Matrix*, 1999

I rushed home, opened the package, read the instructions and talked with Mary. After taking a pill, and waiting the recommended thirty to sixty minutes, I imagined a conversation among my body parts.

Penis: There's too much pressure to perform. Where's the romance?

Rectum: Not like the old days, eh, Penis?

Penis: Those were the days. Standing on command and throughout the night.

Rectum: Well, that's a bit of an exaggeration . . . But you are making improvements.

Penis: Used to be all I needed to hear were the words 'come and get it' and I was good to go.

Rectum: Stay focused, Penis, and don't get discouraged. Stay positive.

Penis: You're right. We promised Prostate we would enjoy life to the fullest. Besides, there's more to life than a mere erection.

At first, my penis was extremely sensitive to the touch, and it didn't take long to reach orgasm, even without an erection. The feeling was incredibly satisfying: more intense and longer-lasting than before the surgery. The only issue was that it was painful at the end of orgasm, and I leaked a bit of urine. However, I was thrilled to achieve this significant milestone.

I found that the pain and leakage[23] gradually diminished and eventually disappeared over time, with practice and patience. As a matter of fact, in one of our private interludes, I experienced something new, something that I had thought only women had the pleasure of enjoying. For the first time in my life, I experienced multiple orgasms. I attribute this to my newfound mindset on making a connection with love and intimacy and keeping in mind that the most important body organ for sex is the brain.[24]

By the sixth month, our sex life had improved dramatically, not just because erections were returning, but because of my new focus on romance, intimacy and love. At first, it was tough to accept that erections were

---

23   If the external sphincter is intact, strong and not damaged, it will remain closed and therefore not allow urine to escape during sex.

24   Having a healthy, loving relationship is a precursor for intimacy, and without the brain to interpret sensations, you'd have no idea you had an orgasm — or any feelings at all, for that matter. Stroking your partner's mind in the right way will go a long way in leading to action.

not as spontaneous as before surgery, but the rewards of building a robust, healthy, loving relationship far outweighed this new reality.

After 17 months of patience and practice, my erections are almost back to normal, although not quite as good as before the surgery. Chances are excellent for a full recovery, though, and eventually I will no longer need the help of the blue pills. Whenever I have trouble, the trick is to remind myself to slow down, and that erections are not the goal. I focus my efforts on making a connection with love. This approach works wonders, and I highly endorse it.

Thinking about erections, I would have appreciated being made aware of the potential risk of losing penis length. Seeing the difference was quite a shock, especially since I had not been told about the possibility. It reminded me of the *Seinfeld* episode where George Costanza yells out, "I was in the pool!"

Jerry: Do women know about shrinkage?

Elaine: What do you mean, like laundry?

Jerry: No, like when a man goes swimming . . . After wards . . .

Elaine: It shrinks?

Jerry: Like a frightened turtle!

Elaine: Why does it shrink?

George: It just does.

Elaine: I don't know how you guys walk around with those things.

— Dialogue from TV series *Seinfeld*, "The Hamptons" episode, 1994

The American Cancer Society suggests that shrinkage is to do with the nerves that control erections. Since these nerves control blood flow, the penis is likely to be smaller until the nerves recover and blood flow returns to normal levels.

An article in *Men's Health* supports this concept, while citing recent MRI studies that seem to show that in some cases, the urethra may move inward towards the pelvis after surgery, taking the penis along with it. However, in most cases, the connective tissues holding the pelvic organs in place generally loosen over time and return to their original position.

Dr. Peter Scardino[25] supports the idea that penis length, either flaccid or erect, depends mostly on blood flow controlled by the erection nerves. Long-lasting nerve damage may lead to atrophy of the vascular channels of the penis, and the fibrous tissue may not expand like it used to before surgery, thus causing penis shortening and not-so-firm erections. Other causes of a shorter-looking penis may include weight gain,[26] Peyronie's disease,[27] aging,[28] and the lack of nighttime erections[29]. He disagrees with the concept of the urethra pulling the penis inside the body like a retracted hose.

---

25 *Dr. Peter Scardino's Prostate Book: The Complete Guide to Overcoming Prostate Cancer, Prostatitis, and BPH*, under "Penis Size and Shape."

26 A visual effect that makes the penis appear shorter.

27 Scar tissue or plaque that forms inside the penis, resulting in a loss of length and a bent erection.

28 Men may lose penis length as they age, due to atrophy, a decline in testosterone and reduced sexual activity.

29 Nighttime erections are essential to stretch the penis, keeping it in shape for action.

(I'm sure a lot of men, including me, would love this concept to be true. You could just retract when not in use, and when needed, simply pull out to the desired length.) Fortunately, for me, the length improved over time, although I've never measured to be sure.

In any case, it's best to be aware of this potential risk and ask your health-care team about it.

CHAPTER NINE

MOVING FORWARD

> Running water never grows stale. So you just have to 'keep on flowing.'
> — Bruce Lee

> There are many ways of going forward, but only one way of standing still.
> — Franklin D. Roosevelt

> Life is like riding a bicycle. To keep your balance, you must keep moving.
> — Albert Einstein

POST-SURGERY MONITORING

EVEN THOUGH THE PATHOLOGY REPORT indicated negative surgical margins and I required no further treatment, I still get anxious when it's time for a follow-up PSA blood test. The continued testing is a precautionary measure to monitor any rise that might suggest prostate cancer cells have been left behind during surgery.

The urologist informed me I should continue getting tested every three months for the first year. Normally, PSA should go down significantly after surgery and will ideally be undetectable, meaning no evidence of cancer cells found. 'Undetectable' results are based on the sensitivity of the lab. If the test can only measure to X, and no PSA is detected, the results are usually reported as <X,[30] which doesn't necessarily mean zero, as it's possible PSA remains at a level less than X.

The urologist explained that any rise in future tests to detectable levels could indicate the cancer is returning. Since the prostate is the only organ that produces PSA, any rise without a prostate suggests[31] that there are still prostate cancer cells in the body that escaped and survived treatment. Over time, these cells can multiply, spread, and produce enough PSA to become detectable. Therefore, after any treatment, it's critical to continue PSA testing for the rest of your life, using the same lab if possible.

In addition to regular PSA testing, it's important not to wait until your next scheduled appointment to report any new signs or symptoms that may have developed since treatment. Symptoms of recurrent prostate cancer vary and may include,

---

30 The < symbol represents "less than." Therefore, <X, reads, "less than X."

31 Since it's possible for normal prostate cells to remain after any treatment, your PSA results become the benchmark to monitor any rise.

- pain or stiffness in the hip, back or chest bones
- loss of sensation or muscle strength in the legs
- loss of bladder control
- a persistent cough
- shortness of breath
- blood in the urine or anus
- pain in the rectum

Prostate cancer recurrence is highest within the first five years,[32] and close attention is required during this time. If cancer has spread outside the prostate, it most likely will develop in nearby lymph nodes and seminal vesicles before travelling to the bones and other organs. Therefore, if your pathology report indicates negative surgical margins, chances are good it hasn't spread beyond the tissue removed. However, it's always best to err on the side of caution and report anything out of the ordinary to your health-care team.

As a matter of fact, on July 4, 2018, I woke up in the middle of the night with intense lower back pain directly over my spine that wouldn't go away. It was an 8 out of 10 on the pain scale. After I took some pain medication and applied Voltaren, the pain subsided in about 20 minutes. Therefore, I wasn't sure if this was bone pain or muscle pain. The next day, I felt fine. However, once again, the pain returned during the night.

---

32 That said, please note that it's not unusual for recurrence to occur much later, even ten or more years after treatment.

After the fourth night, being stressed about cancer recurrence, I made an appointment with my family doctor and reported it to my urologist, who ordered another PSA test.

After my doctor examined my back, she set up a CT scan. I'm happy to report that the CT scan found no evidence of metastatic disease, and PSA was undetectable. The night pain was most likely due to my having strained a back muscle while doing heavy yard work a few days before.

Since the surgery, I've had five PSA blood tests. All showed results of <0.008, or undetectable. The urologist has now reduced the frequency of the test to every six months for the next three years. If the results continue to be undetectable, the frequency will be reduced to once a year.

In the unlikely event my PSA results were to rise to detectable levels, I've been advised to monitor the situation and consider further treatment only if levels rise above 0.2 ng/ml. Of course, I am to continue to keep my urologist updated with any concerns.

If you opt for radiation over surgery, it's normal for PSA to rise and fall over the next two years. After that, you may need to consider further treatment options if PSA rises by 2.0 ng/ml or more above the lowest reading over those two years.

Celebration Cruise Mishap

To celebrate the success of my surgery of just five months previous, Mary and I booked a cruise-and-stay package to Disneyland. The cruise was scheduled to depart from Vancouver on October 1, 2017, and sail down the California coast for five nights, stopping at Astoria, Santa Barbara, San Francisco and Los Angeles. We would stay in Anaheim for four nights to visit Disneyland and Universal Studios, then end the trip with a flight home on October 11.

I strongly urge you, too, to get away after your treatment if possible, to get back into life.

We looked forward to the celebration.

However, unfortunately, a few months before our trip, Mary tripped on uneven concrete in our backyard while changing the nectar in the hummingbird feeder. It was quite upsetting to hear Alex call: "Dad! Mom fell — come quick!" I rushed out to the backyard and kneeled by her side to assess the situation. Mary was dazed and confused, and her left wrist was dreadfully swollen.

Gogs: Mary, what happened? Are you all right?
Mary: I don't know, but I'm fine.
Gogs: Let's get you to emergency, just to be sure.
Mary: No, it's all right, just give me a minute.

Mary's altruistic nature makes her an excellent caregiver, but not necessarily the best patient. She follows her mother's philosophy of always putting the needs of others before her own. She was concerned that her injury wouldn't be as important as others' in the emergency room. But it was my turn to look after her.

Although an X-ray didn't reveal any broken bones, there was a widening between some of the bones in her wrist, so Mary was referred to a plastic surgeon for a second opinion on treatment. About a month later, we met with the plastic surgeon, who examined her wrist and didn't see the need for any treatment, telling us that everything should heal on its own. That was a relief, as we were looking forward to our upcoming trip.

Over the next few months, Mary continued to have pain. However, she insisted that under no circumstances was she going to cancel or postpone our celebration cruise.

Mary: We're going, and don't worry about me. I'll be fine, and besides, you need time away to help with your recovery.

Again, thinking of others' needs over her own.

She was convincing. On October 1, we boarded the cruise ship at Canada Place in Vancouver. By and large, it was a wonderful trip, filled with adventure and fun, although Mary continued to have wrist pain. Being a trouper, she rarely complained and even insisted we go on all the rides at Disneyland and Universal Studios.

After our trip, there was still no significant improvement. Mary continued to be in pain and had difficulty coping with daily tasks. This was disappointing, as we had thought things should be a whole lot better after all this time.

Finally, a CT scan on December 5 revealed a severe fracture of her scaphoid bone. This untreated fracture was the reason for all the pain and suffering Mary had endured since her fall almost four months before.

Two days later, a bone-and-joint specialist successfully performed a left proximal row removal of three carpal bones and rebuilt her wrist with the remaining bones. A few weeks later, we had a follow-up visit with the specialist. He removed the cast and wrappings from her wrist to reveal a five-inch incision, which surprised us — we hadn't expected it to be so long. However, the wrist looked great and was no longer swollen.

Mary breathed a sigh of relief as she carefully moved her wrist about while experiencing little or no pain. I held her other hand while we kissed to celebrate the success.

It was clear the specialist was also delighted with the results, as we heard him laugh out loud. He predicted that Mary would regain total mobility of her wrist, which was music to our ears.

We thanked him and went out for a celebration dinner.

Reflection and Final Thoughts

Being diagnosed with prostate cancer was a total shock that caught my family and me completely off guard. It hit us so hard that we were stunned for many months, and we're still a bit dazed to this day. The whole experience was life-altering. It has forced us to re-evaluate our priorities and values moving forward. Even though it was challenging at times, changing our mindset to focus on the positives helped us tremendously to cope throughout my diagnosis, surgery and recovery.

The American Cancer Society and the Canadian Cancer Society estimate that for 2019, in the US and Canada alone, approximately 195,950 men (174,650 American, 21,300 Canadian) will be diagnosed with prostate cancer, of which roughly 35,720 men (31,620 American, 4,100 Canadian) will die from the disease. On average, that's almost 537 North American men diagnosed with — and nearly 98 who will die from — the disease every single day in 2019 (that's about one man every 15 minutes).

The lifetime probability for men to develop prostate cancer in Canada is 1 in 7, while in America it's 1 in 9.

The best hope for successful prostate cancer treatment and recovery is early-stage detection. Prostate cancer can be deadly when it reaches more advanced stages. However, because the disease usually doesn't have any early symptoms, routine testing is essential.

Readers should note that I had no noticeable symptoms of any kind. Even several digital rectal examinations by different doctors over a five-year period reported everything to be smooth and normal.

Therefore, without the PSA tests that identified rising results, followed by an MRI that identified an abnormal area, followed by a targeted prostate biopsy, I wouldn't have known about my cancer — especially the fact that it was already in the final stage before extending outside the prostate.

Since I was 57 years old at the time, it most likely would have spread outside the prostate within my lifetime. The chances of a full recovery at that point would have been much smaller. There would have been a higher possibility of death from the cancer, along with an increased risk of permanent side effects from the treatment.

Even though the PSA test helped me significantly, please be aware that there is controversy surrounding the test, which does produce many false positive and false negative results. In other words, an elevated PSA doesn't necessarily mean you have cancer, and a low PSA doesn't necessarily mean you don't.

False-positive elevated PSA results can lead to unnecessary anxiety and unnecessary biopsies, with the risk of bleeding, pain, infection, temporary urinary difficulties and other issues. Remember, my PSA was monitored over five years and was measured 14 times. Its disturbing upward trend made a better case for an MRI and a targeted prostate biopsy.

Even though I opted for surgery, there are many other treatment options to consider, depending on your test results and situation. Because no single treatment is best for everyone, it's essential to be aware of the alternatives before making a final decision. In fact, you have lots of options to discuss with your health-care team, including, in alphabetical order,

- active surveillance (regular testing, PSA, DRE, MRI, various scans and biopsies)
- chemotherapy (drugs)
- cryosurgery (freezing)
- HIFU, high-intensity focused ultrasound (burning)
- hormone therapy (androgen deprivation therapy [ADT], androgen suppression therapy [AST])
- immunotherapies (monoclonal antibodies, immune checkpoint inhibitors, cancer vaccines)
- radiation therapy (external beam,[33] brachytherapy[34])
- radical prostatectomy (open, laparoscopic, robotic)
- transurethral resection of the prostate (TURP)
- and many different forms or combinations of the above, including a variety of medications.

An increasingly popular option is genetic and genomic testing.

---

33 There are many forms of external beam radiation therapy, such as three-dimensional conformal (3D-CRT), intensity-modulated (IMRT), volumetric-modulated arc (VMAT), image-guided (IGRT), stereotactic body (SBRT) and proton beam. Often these treatments are known by the names of the machines that deliver the radiation, such as linear accelerator (LINAC), CyberKnife and Gamma Knife.

34 There are two forms of brachytherapy: permanent (low-dose rate, or LDR) and temporary implant (high-dose rate, or HDR).

Genetics looks for mutations in the BRCA genes that are passed on from generation to generation. These genes repair cell damage, and if they contain abnormalities, you're at a higher risk to develop prostate cancer.

Knowing you have a higher risk would support the need for more regular PSA and DRE tests as you age.

Genomic testing predicts tumour aggressiveness by looking at specific genes within the tumour tissue to report if the cancer is a low, medium or high risk and how likely it is to grow and spread. Knowing your results can help with the treatment decision.

Since these tests are always evolving, it's best to consult with your health-care team for the latest developments.

Above all, living a healthy and active lifestyle may slow down the growth of prostate cancer, or lower the risk of it coming back after treatment. I'm sure all those years eating junk food didn't help my situation.

As an afterthought, all of my post-diagnosis research focused on treatment options, with zero time spent on healthy eating. Even though my urologist provided information on nutrition, I mostly ignored it and made changes on my own without research or support. Big mistake. Improving your diet should be the first step in any treatment option, and it requires serious effort and commitment.

Generally speaking, for cancer contained within the prostate, all options can be considered.

However, treatment options potentially become more limited as cancer spreads further outside the prostate. If no option is suitable for personal or medical reasons, or a treatment has failed to produce the desired results, there are always new treatments on the horizon. Ask your health-care team about clinical trials to keep on top of the latest developments.

I now believe that I dismissed radiation options too quickly. I did so because I was concerned that if radiation failed to destroy all cancer cells, surgery would no longer be an option, or would at least be more complex[35] for the surgeon. Also, since I had experienced a few major operations already — all with positive results and fond memories — I was fine with the idea of another surgery. Even so, these reasons were certainly not justification for dismissing radiation or other treatment options without giving them fair consideration.

Please take time with your decision and keep an open mind. Sometimes we tend to blind ourselves by being too focused on what we think is right, without taking enough time to look at other options. After all,

---

35   Surgery can be more complicated because radiation can cause fibrosis (scarring), which can make it difficult for the surgeon to distinguish the bladder from the prostate from the rectum, as these organs are somewhere in the scar tissue. In contrast, radiation after surgery is more straightforward, since a CT scan can localize the intended target and bypass the fibrosis to get directly to the cancer. Either way, please note that surgery also causes fibrosis and therefore all second treatment options carry an increased risk of complication.

it's your body, and it deserves your time. Also, please don't be pressured one way or another. All treatment options can be viable, depending on your situation, and besides, it's a personal choice. Think about what matters to you.

If there were only one thing I could do differently, it would be to join a support group with Mary before making the final decision to have surgery. There are both online and brick-and-mortar support groups available, and I encourage you to join several. In general, I prefer the social aspect of meeting others face to face. I find the interaction very bonding. However, no matter the source of your support, recognize that each case is different, and not everyone will experience the same outcomes. Even though my results have been very positive, they could have been very negative. In that case, I would have regretted surgery and kicked myself for not having joined a support group earlier. Not only would it have potentially given us more options to research, but it might also have better prepared us for surgery and dealing with potential side effects. At the very least, we would have made new friends who shared a special bond.

However, it's never too late to join. We attended our first support-group meeting in May of 2018. Even one year after the surgery, it gave us a sense of camaraderie to know we were not alone. We found it encouraging and inspiring to have the opportunity to listen and speak to other men and their loved ones in similar situations. I had always thought that asking for help was a sign of weakness, but I have since learned that notion couldn't be further from the truth. There's strength in numbers. The more people helping, the stronger you become as you learn from their experience, which is extremely valuable.

Depending on where you live, I highly recommend connecting with both a local group and one from a larger city — it's worth considering driving to a larger group, even if it's only once or twice a year. The Comox Valley support group is small, and services are limited, so in July we visited the BC Cancer clinic at the Royal Jubilee Hospital in Victoria. We were very impressed. The clinic offers a comprehensive survivorship program for men with prostate cancer and their partners and families. This program provides support with treatment-decision-making, rehabilitation needs post-treatment and lifestyle management, including nutrition and exercise. Counselling services are available, as well as an extensive library of books, videos and CDs.

At 21 months post-surgery, my PSA remains undetectable, meaning there is no evidence of cancer cells left behind during surgery and no further treatment is required at this time.

As a matter of interest, two weeks after surgery, I experienced quite a bit of numbness in my lower back that was due to the spinal anesthetic injected by the anesthesiologist, who had warned me of a small risk of permanent nerve damage. However, within six months, the numbness had completely disappeared.

The best news is that I have had no lasting side effects. Incontinence lasted six weeks and erections started to return after three months, and after 17 months were firm enough for intercourse. However, please be aware that each case is different, and results will vary significantly depending on your current health, age, family history, present urinary control, existing erection quality, surgeon, skill and experience, how far cancer invaded your body, and many other factors.

Even though I've had a very successful recovery and am almost back to 100 percent, many men do not recover fully, regardless of the treatment they choose. Many men lose interest in sex, never regain erectile function, or suffer from continued urinary incontinence. There are many other risks of treatment that in some extremely rare cases may include death (if you have pre-existing heart disease or other serious health problems).

Please talk to your doctor and ask questions. There are many support, and couples' therapy groups that you can join even before you decide on treatment. Research as much as possible. Talk with other cancer survivors, family and friends, and more than one doctor.

In my experience, the more I learned, the more empowered I felt. And the more I shared with others, the more I was able to accept the situation, clear my mind and make a decision. The winning factor for me was that I had a great deal of confidence and trust in my surgeon and his team, which allowed me to move forward with surgery and to focus energy and strength on recovery. I was of the mindset that even if side effects were permanent and surgery failed to remove all cancer, it wouldn't be the end of the world, and certainly not the end of my happiness. There are far too many things in life to be grateful for, even without an erection or with having to wear a pad.

The whole experience gave us a new appreciation and respect for life. It brought us closer as a family, and we learned to slow down and treasure every moment. One thing that helped me cope throughout was to realize that being diagnosed with prostate cancer was not only tough for me but it was also tough for my loved ones. They, too, needed to be part of the process.

Since it's possible for a few prostate cancer cells to remain undetected in the body after any treatment, it's vital to continue to live an active, healthy lifestyle, with regular PSA testing. That said, please don't stress over this fact. It's not necessary to hear the words "no evidence of disease" to live a happy and meaningful life. Even when the prognosis is not good, sometimes hope lies in the unknown. In the event of recurrence where subsequent treatments are unsuitable or have failed, hope always exists as there are several drugs available, and new ones in development, to help manage prostate cancer for a long time.

For recovery, my goal is to be healthier and stronger than I was before surgery. Since I moved to the Comox Valley, my activity levels have dropped significantly, as I no longer ride my bike to work, train in the work gym or train with my karate buddies. After three years of basically little activity, and the return to eating junk food after surgery, I've finally decided to get back into the gym. Even though I'm no stranger to exercise, my long absence required starting at the beginning.

In June 2018, just over one year post-surgery, I hired a personal trainer and nutritionist to get me back on track. I'm confident I'll be able to work hard in the gym, although giving up junk food won't be easy. But now I'm armed with the awareness that when I reach for treats, I'm really reaching for fond memories of childhood. Knowing and remembering this fact should help break the habit. Also, it simply makes sense to follow a healthy diet and engage in physical exercise to help reduce the risk of developing cancer and other health issues.

It's never too late to embrace healthy living. There's plenty of information available on becoming active and healthy from books, the internet, and medical professionals. A simple test to help determine if you're overweight is to divide waist size by height. The results should be less than 50 percent, or in other words, ideally, your waist should be less than half your height. Check with your health-care team to determine what's right for you.

Mary, too, is on the road to a full recovery after her unfortunate fall and broken wrist. Since her wrist surgery, she has made remarkable progress and has regained complete mobility. She only experiences minor pain on occasions, and although she still has numbness, it's slowly improving. Mary also has a goal to be healthier and stronger. She has started a walking program with a friend and enjoys swimming.

Life isn't about waiting for the storm to pass. It's about learning how to dance in the rain.

— Vivian Greene

A final few words on being diagnosed with prostate cancer. The first thing is: don't panic. It didn't pop up overnight. Most likely it has been in the prostate for a long time already, perhaps years, and is only now big enough to be detected. Even if it's fairly aggressive, prostate cancer grows slowly compared to other cancers. Therefore, don't think the worst. It's better to detect cancer than to overlook it. The good news is that treatments have improved significantly over the years. There are many options available and always breakthroughs on the horizon. This includes not only new treatment breakthroughs but also new and more sensitive imaging, such as the PET (positron emission tomography) scan, that may more precisely identify prostate cancer metastases[36] in the body over traditional bone and CT scans.

Next, take a breath and realize that you're not alone. There are literally millions of other people affected by prostate cancer. It's essential to share your feelings with family, friends and your health-care team. Be open and honest about your feelings and engage in healthy discussions.

---

36   Cancer cells that have spread to another part of the body from where the cancer first started.

You may find that some of your friends or family tend to avoid you, and that's okay. Sometimes they don't know how to respond, or they could be going through troubling times of their own. Many of them may return later, once they've had time to process. But you may also find that casual acquaintances become strong supporters, or you may even unexpectedly make new friends. All of this happened to me, and I couldn't be happier. Although I've lost touch with a few friends, many of my old childhood buddies, relatives, colleagues and neighbours have surfaced to provide encouragement and kind words when I needed them most.

Reach out to support groups and speak to others who have gone before you. Sharing your story will benefit others and give you the opportunity to get things off your mind. It's important not to blame yourself for the cancer and struggle with the "Why me?" question, as this will only add to your stress. Instead of beating yourself up, it's much better to focus on dealing with the issue. Being gentle with yourself and learning how to live a healthy lifestyle by eating nutritious foods, exercising and reducing stress will not only help prevent your cancer from getting worse, it will also help keep you from developing heart disease, diabetes and other cancers.

Above all, give yourself at least enough time to recover from the initial shock of your diagnosis before making a decision. Become your own health advocate and understand your test results. Research your options based on the best available evidence from scientific research, reputable studies and facts. Even the best medical professionals in the world are human. They're capable of making mistakes. Some may even have their own self-interests in mind. Or they may be limited by their own modality, so that a radiation oncologist may endorse radiation while a surgeon may prescribe surgery.

If possible, bring someone with you to all your appointments and have them take notes while you ask questions from a list you prepared ahead of time. Don't be afraid to ask for more than one opinion or travel to a larger city that has a centre that specializes in prostate cancer. Asking for other opinions relates not only to treatment options but also to confirming if your diagnosis is correct. It's far better to take your time than to rush into treatment and later regret it.

Although all treatment options can be very successful, especially in early-stage diagnosis, the harsh reality is that not everyone will survive cancer. It's always a good idea to ensure your affairs are in order, and that your loved ones understand and will honour your last wishes.

If you are about to begin treatment (other than active surveillance) and are not yet retired, please plan to take time off work for recovery. Depending on your type of work and the procedure, you may need anywhere from a few days to several weeks. I found six weeks away from the office was extremely beneficial to my health.

Completing treatment can be both stressful and exciting. It's most likely a relief, but fears of possible recurrence can be hard to avoid. Therefore, it's critical to celebrate the end of treatment. It's a significant milestone that deserves recognition. Find a way to take pleasure in this momentous occasion, regardless of the unknown future.

In fact, it's far more rewarding to celebrate every milestone than to ignore them. Throw a party. Invite friends. Enjoy life!

Depression and fatigue are possible side effects of prostate cancer treatment, which can make it even harder to find the motivation to improve diet and engage in physical activity. This is another good reason to connect with a support group — to look for inspiration and realize you're not alone. Reach out to the community, develop new hobbies or interests and look for ways to improve your overall health, including your mind, body and soul.

That said, please recognize recovery will not be overnight. In fact, don't overdo it like I did the first day in the gym a year after surgery. (My mind was ready, but my body disagreed.) After 45 minutes of working out with my personal trainer, Michelle, I started to lose vision and was close to blacking out. She started escorting me to a nearby chair, but I collapsed to the floor along the way. After a couple of juice boxes and a long talk, my energy returned. This was not simply due to the sugar but also to the professionalism and support of my trainer. She was inspirational, motivational and full of great advice regarding nutrition and healthy living.

I had pushed too hard without even realizing it, my mind too busy reminiscing over the glory years of my youth. With Michelle's help and counsel, I've accepted my new level and have since been making good progress in the gym. If possible, I highly suggest hiring a personal trainer and not going it alone.

Although it may be hard to accept your new life — particularly dealing with the potential side effects of treatment — it's best to stay positive and find alternative paths to your goals.

No matter which treatment you decide on, from active surveillance to more invasive options, I wish you the very best outcome and that you live a long, healthy and fulfilling life.

In the words of Spock from *Star Trek*, "Live long and prosper".

What day is it?" asked Pooh.
"It's today," squeaked Piglet.
"My favourite day," said Pooh.

— A. A. Milne, *Winnie the Pooh*

Bibliography

Books

BC Cancer Agency
Nutrition Guide for Men with Prostate Cancer
2016

Ellsworth, Pamela
100 Questions & Answers about Prostate Cancer, 5th ed.
Burlington, MA: Jones & Bartlett Learning, 2018

Goldenberg, S. Larry; Pickles, Tom; and Chi, Kim N.
The Intelligent Patient Guide to Prostate Cancer, 4th ed.
Intelligent Patient Guide, 2014

Scardino, Peter
Dr. Peter Scardino's Prostate Book: The Complete Guide to Overcoming Prostate Cancer, Prostatitis, and BPH, 2nd ed.
New York: Avery, 2010

Servan-Schreiber, David
Anticancer: A New Way of Life
New York: Penguin Random House, 2017

Walsh, Patrick and Farrar Worthington, Janet
Dr. Patrick Walsh's Guide to Surviving Prostate Cancer, 4th ed.
Grand Central Life & Style, 2018

Websites – Prostate Cancer Testing

Bone scan - Canadian Cancer Society
https://www.cancer.ca/en/cancer-information/diagnosis-and-treatment/tests-and-procedures/bone-scan/?region=bc

CT (computed tomography) scan - Canadian Cancer Society
https://www.cancer.ca/en/cancer-information/diagnosis-and-treatment/tests-and-procedures/computed-tomography-ct-scan/?region=bc

Cystoscopy - Canadian Cancer Society
https://www.cancer.ca/en/cancer-information/diagnosis-and-treatment/tests-and-procedures/cystoscopy/?region=bc

Echocardiogram (Echo) - Canadian Cancer Society
https://www.cancer.ca/en/cancer-information/diagnosis-and-treatment/tests-and-procedures/echocardiogram/?region=bc

Electrocardiogram (ECG) - Canadian Cancer Society
https://www.cancer.ca/en/cancer-information/diagnosis-and-treatment/tests-and-procedures/electrocardiogram-ecg/?region=bc

MRI (magnetic resonance imaging) scan - Canadian Cancer Society
https://www.cancer.ca/en/cancer-information/diagnosis-and-treatment/tests-and-procedures/magnetic-resonance-imaging-mri/?region=bc

Prostate biopsy - About - Mayo Clinic
https://www.mayoclinic.org/tests-procedures/prostate-biopsy/about/pac-20384734

PSA (prostate-specific antigen) test - National Cancer Institute
https://www.cancer.gov/types/prostate/psa-fact-sheet#q3

PSA levels during and after prostate cancer treatment - American Cancer Society
https://www.cancer.org/cancer/prostate-cancer/treating/psa-levels-after-treatment.html

PSA rising - Prostate Cancer Foundation
https://www.pcf.org/about-prostate-cancer/diagnosis-staging-prostate-cancer/psa-rising

WEBSITES – PROSTATE CANCER TREATMENTS

Active surveillance for prostate cancer - Canadian Cancer Society
https://www.cancer.ca/en/cancer-information/cancer-type/prostate/treatment/active-surveillance/?region=bc

Brachytherapy therapy (internal radiation) - Canadian Cancer Society
https://www.cancer.ca/en/cancer-information/diagnosis-and-treatment/radiation-therapy/internal-radiation-therapy/?region=bc4

Chemotherapy for prostate cancer - Canadian Cancer Society
https://www.cancer.ca/en/cancer-information/cancer-type/prostate/treatment/chemotherapy/?region=bc

Cryosurgery - Canadian Cancer Society

https://www.cancer.ca/en/cancer-information/diagnosis-and-treatment/tests-and-procedures/cryosurgery/?region=bc

External beam radiation therapy - Canadian Cancer Society

https://www.cancer.ca/en/cancer-information/diagnosis-and-treatment/radiation-therapy/external-radiation-therapy/?region=bc

HIFU (high-intensity focused ultrasound) - Prostate Cancer Canada

http://www.prostatecancer.ca/Prostate-Cancer/Treatment/High-Intensity-Focused-Ultrasound-(HIFU)

Hormonal therapy for prostate cancer - Canadian Cancer Society

https://www.cancer.ca/en/cancer-information/cancer-type/prostate/treatment/hormonal-therapy/?region=bc

Radiation therapy for prostate cancer - Canadian Cancer Society

https://www.cancer.ca/en/cancer-information/cancer-type/prostate/treatment/radiation-therapy/?region=bc

Surgery for prostate cancer - Canadian Cancer Society

https://www.cancer.ca/en/cancer-information/cancer-type/prostate/treatment/surgery/?region=bc

Systemic radiation therapy - American Cancer Society

https://www.cancer.org/treatment/treatments-and-side-effects/treatment-types/radiation/systemic-radiation-therapy.html

Websites – Research

American Cancer Society
http://www.cancer.org

BC Cancer Clinic
http://www.bccancer.bc.ca/

Canadian Cancer Society
https://www.cancer.ca

Mayo Clinic
http://www.mayoclinic.org

National Cancer Institute
http://www.cancer.gov

Prostate Cancer Canada
http://www.prostatecancer.ca

Prostate Cancer Foundation
http://www.pcf.org

Prostate Cancer Foundation BC
http://www.prostatecancerbc.ca

Vancouver Prostate Centre
http://www.prostatecentre.com

Websites – Support Groups

American Cancer Society
https://www.cancer.org/treatment/support-programs-and-services.html

Prostate Cancer Canada
http://www.prostatecancer.ca/Support/Services/Support-Groups

Prostate Cancer Foundation
https://www.pcf.org/c/finding-a-support-group

CONNECTING WITH GOGS

You may contact Gogs through one of his social media sites or leave him a review on Amazon. He sincerely thanks you for reading.

Facebook Author Page
https://www.facebook.com/OfficialGogsGagnon

Twitter
https://twitter.com/GogsGagnon

Website
https://GogsGagnon.com/

YouTube
https://www.youtube.com/c/GogsGagnon

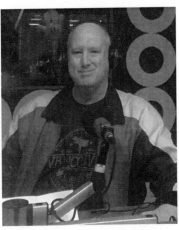

Gogs Gagnon at the CKNW studio
in Vancouver, BC.

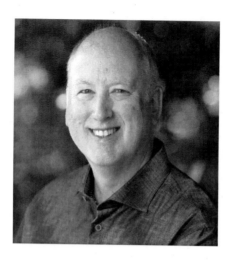

A native of New Westminster, **Gogs Gagnon** followed an early passion for computers by becoming a programmer and independent technology consultant. In the course of his career, he has developed software for Apple, IBM, and the government of British Columbia, where he was the lead programmer analyst and data architect.

Now, in addition to promoting prostate cancer awareness, Gogs devotes much of his time to writing. His next book is a coming-of-age novel set in the Lower Mainland of British Columbia during the 1970s.

The father of three children, Gogs lives with his wife and their two dogs in the Comox Valley on Vancouver Island, BC.